Men and Their Emotions
Anxiety, Fear, Anger and
The relationship With Your Penis...................32
    Sexual Desire......................35
The Health of Emotions.................37
The Emotional Nature of Sex................41
Performance Anxiety: A Self-Fulfilling Prophecy.............42
For the single man.................44
The Solution: A Team Effort.................46
Maintaining Arousal.................49
Identifying and Naming Your Feelings.............52
    Emotions.................52
    Fear and Anxiety.................54
    Avoidance.................55
    Anger.................55
    Staying in the Present.................58
Importance of Relationship Connection.............59
Teammates, Friends and Lovers.................64
The Rigors of Relating.................67
For the Partner.................69
    For the Partner in Relating.................72
A Man's Relationship with Himself.................74
    Loving Yourself.................76
    Integrity.................78
    Responsibility and Ownership.................79
    The King and the Queen.................80
Letting Go.................81
    Pressure and Force.................83
    One-Way Thinking.................84
    Control.................84
Contributing Factors.................86
    Sexual Factors.................87
    Past Abuse.................88
    Ejaculatory Control Problems.................89
    Discrepancy of Sexual Desire.................92
    Desire.................93

Orgasm	94
Vaginismus	95
Penis Size	96
Non-Sexual Contributing Factors	99
Goal Orientation	99
Trying	100
The Worker Being Productive	101
Playfulness	102
Medications	103
Let Sex Be a Strength	105
Setting Yourself Up for Success	112
Index of exercises	115

Course Instructions: *While the focus of this course is on the man who has had challenges maintaining his erection, if a female partner is in his life, her support will be essential. This course is for all men in either heterosexual or homosexual relationships. However, throughout the text, language of heterosexual relationships will be used. The man stuck in the performance anxiety cycle will have to do most of the work, but this course will be most effective if the partner participates throughout. Success will benefit both of you. Some instructions are included for a single man. Throughout the course are exercises which include writing a journal, reflecting, discussing and an audio relaxation exercise. The potential for success is maximized if these are performed regularly and diligently. Significant time and effort may have to be devoted to the goal for your success to be achieved.*

Note of Caution: *We must be certain that your experience of erection loss is not caused by a physical condition. For this book to be useful for you, the source of your erection problems must be emotionally-based. In the past month do you ever have a lasting erection (at least 3-5 minutes)? Do you have erections when you masturbate? Do you have partial or soft erections? Take some time and experiment with masturbation. If you answered "no" to all these questions, consult with a physician before continuing with the remainder of this book.*

What is the Problem?

Performance anxiety is a vicious cycle in which a man fears that he will be unable to perform sexually, by failing to maintain his erection long enough to satisfy his female partner. Within the challenge of performance anxiety, is that if a man fears failure, then he does fail. The

> Performance Anxiety: if a man fears failure, then he will fail.

cycle is energized by a man's escalating emotion, most commonly the emotion of fear. For good sexual functioning and sexual success, a man requires confidence. The cycle of performance anxiety undermines a man's confidence in having and maintaining an erection when he wants it the most; when he has an available sexual partner who he strongly wishes to satisfy.

For men, sex is a primal activity that flows from the core of their masculine being. A man's ability to attract a partner and engage sexually with her is of vital importance to prove his masculine worthiness and to fulfill what many men feel is a vital male obligation: to succeed sexually and satisfy his partner. Failure to accomplish this casts doubt on a man's masculine worthiness. Men who fail sexually are saddled with painful feelings of inadequacy; they worry that they are not "man enough." Being sexually successful is of supreme importance to men. The importance of success is one contributing factor in the seemingly impossible problem of the cycle of performance anxiety.

Emotional exercise 1: Think about the two preceding paragraphs. By yourself or with your partner, discuss how true these ideas are for you. Write down the conclusion of your thoughts or discussion. Keep the answers to the exercises in a journal where you will regularly record your thoughts, feelings, experiences and observations while you proceed in this course. On my website, helpforpassion.com, you may download a 13-minute audio relaxation exercise for free. It is free by entering the coupon code: FREETORELAX. Listen to this exercise at least once daily and follow the instructions I give by voice. Just this relaxation exercise alone has helped some men overcome erectile dysfunction and performance anxiety.

Sexual exercise 1: Temporarily discontinue intercourse during sexual experiences. You and your sexual partner may engage in sex as often as the two of you like and enjoy pleasuring each other in every possible way **except** for intercourse. The ban on intercourses will last until you feel more confident, which may be from one to three weeks, depending upon how well you practice the course suggestions. Experiment with new ways to give and receive sexual pleasure but stay away from intercourse. Do not violate this rule. Discuss this with your female partner. Even if you have a solid, glorious erection, do not engage in intercourse until later in the course. Discontinuing intercourse is encouraged from the beginning of this process and will be re-introduced once your chance of success has increased. Record your experiences of arousal regularly in your journal.

How does it manifest?

Performance Anxiety is also often referred to as Erectile Dysfunction (ED). The difference between the two names is that erectile dysfunction refers to the result of the problem, erection loss, whereas performance anxiety refers to the cause, which is anxiety. I prefer to use the term performance anxiety because many factors can cause erection loss whereas anxiety is a specific and singular cause of this problem. Performance anxiety shows up in moments of sexual opportunity when a man both expects and desires to have a fully erect penis and he either does not develop an erection or has an erection and loses it before he wishes. The unfortunate loss occurs before or during intercourse and before his and his female partner's completion. A man who does not fall into the trap of performance anxiety loses his erection during sex, shifts his focus to other kinds of pleasuring, and doesn't think of it again. In the next sexual encounter, his erection is lasting, and he performs well. The man who becomes trapped in the cycle of performance anxiety, however, loses his erection and panics. He then has erection problems in most sexual encounters thereafter. Most men experience a lack of erection at some point in their lives, but the event need not be a crisis.

A result of erection failure for the man trapped in the cycle of performance anxiety is disappointment, frustration, embarrassment, shame, and distrust in himself and his penis. The intensity of the painful experience may loom so large that it creates a painful emotional impression that lasts a long time. For the man who has experienced erection loss at an important moment, such as when he is with a partner who he truly cares for and wishes to impress, the impact of failure fills him with doubt and dread in each sexual experience afterwards. He doubts that he is capable of success and dreads that he will once again fail. For many men upon trying again, they once again fail. With every new failure, the grip of the cycle of performance anxiety grows tighter.

Men routinely react to failure in one way, to try harder. Because of their relationship to strength and power, they automatically use more force and effort in a second attempt. The man may get lucky and produce a good result, but more likely is his inflexible attitude will prove ineffective because his method is insensitive to his emotions, the situation, and his partner. In situations of erection loss, the automatic use of more force and effort typically has tragic results. The trap of performance anxiety grows worse.

Some men experience intermittent failures. They have moments of success or partial success in between sporadic failures. Men who only partially succeed may hide their erection loss by distracting their sexual partner or make excuses that are unrelated to the erection loss. What confuses many men is that they may have successful solid erections during masturbation. The inconsistency of erections seems to make no sense and further erodes a man's confidence because he feels out of control.

Emotional exercise 2: Think back on the times you have maintained your erection and times you have lost your erection. Are these instances consistent or intermittent? What percentage of the time do you have a good erection during masturbation? What percentage of the time do you have a good erection during partner sex? Is there a difference in these percentages? Why do you think this is so? Write down your answers.

Sexual exercise 2: Make time for solo sex. In between partner sexual experiences, arrange for privacy when you will masturbate. During masturbation, recall memories of the most exciting past sexual experiences when with your partner. Keep your partner aware of when you masturbate and the quality of your erections. Doing so is a positive strengthening exercise. Take note in your journal of the quality of erections during masturbation.

How does it affect the man?

The importance of sex to men cannot be understated. Sex is so important that it may consume his purpose, thoughts and focus for phases of his life. Men will override their values and even at times what is in their best interest to obtain sex. In most world cultures, prostitution flourishes to satisfy the male need for sex in spite of

> When a man fails to fulfill what he views as an essential male function, his worth plummets.

significant moral and ethical ambivalence. So when a man fails to fulfill what he views as an essential male function, his worth plummets.

Men who are unable to maintain their erections feel their level of confidence is devastated. The shame and embarrassment they feel is profound. Most men, however, have been socialized to avoid showing weakness and therefore may use all their strength to cover up their inner pain, especially to a female partner. An inner experience of pain but an outward display of strength results in a man who is deeply divided and conflicted. He may feel compelled to continually fake confidence, strength and power to hide his inner self-doubt so that only he and his sexual partner know that he is unable to fulfill a man's basic duty.

As a group, men avoid activities at which they believe they will fail. In what we can call the "Man Code," a set of unwritten rules that dictate male values and behavior, is an imperative need to avoid showing weakness. Men stick to this rule implicitly. Once a man experiences sexual failure due to erection loss, he is likely to avoid sexual opportunities. Doing so may be about hiding his failure. For some men, the dread of failure may become all-consuming. Some male partners discontinue affection for their female partners believing that affection will start the journey towards a sexual experience, which they wish to avoid. Men who are not in relationships stop dating for fear that they will go on a date with a woman who has sexual expectations. Many men who cannot perform believe that the women they date will expect intercourse, even on the first date...sex they cannot provide. The power of the fear of failure is truly amazing. Men with enormous sex drives who are trapped in the cycle of performance anxiety suddenly have no sexual interest. They may even develop a sexual aversion in which they purposefully avoid every sexual opportunity. Female partners of these men are often totally confused by their male partner's sudden shift in sexual attitude.

The longer the inability to be sexually successful lasts, the more shame-ridden a man grows. Some men become obsessed with this problem and ruminate about it constantly, leaving them feeling powerless. Other men inflate the importance of sex so that everything is a reminder of their painful inadequacy. Some fear that their sexual failures will eventually cost them their relationships, their marriages, and their families. Some of these men are right.

How hard is an erection? This is called tumescence, or the degree that a penis or other organ becomes firm when it is engorged with blood. Penis hardness varies from man to man and from age to age. As we age, the maximum hardness of our erections normally decreases. Our erections were more solid at age 16 than at age 45 and harder at 45 than 65. If we have a healthy body, we should be able to have a good enough erection through most of our lives. A good enough erection is one in which penetration for intercourse is possible. Unrealistic expectations of our erections can result in erection failure.

Emotional exercise 3: Reflect on the impact that unreliable or unavailable erections have on you, your feelings, and your self-esteem. How did you react when you first experienced erection failure? Did the uncertainty of your erections change how you felt about sex? In what way? Write down your answers.

Sexual exercise 3: During the past week, how many sexual experiences have you and your partner had? Have you been successful at not engaging in intercourse? How difficult has that been? During your non-intercourse sex, have you had any erections? Record in your journal the qualities of your erections; whether they were reliable, steady, partial, intermittent, or non-existent. Make note of when you had an erection, how hard it was (0-10), and what you have felt at times when your erection was present, most hard or absent. Practice letting go of negative feelings when your penis is not erect.

How Do Your Erection Difficulties Affect Your Partner?

Female partners react to male erectile dysfunction in a wide variety of ways, from supportive to enraged. A woman who is with a man whose erection has just faded is in a bind; express her true painful feelings and undermine the possibility that he will overcome the problem or act gently with compassion and be inauthentic in expressing her disappointment. Most women initially react with fear that their

> Most women initially react with fear that her man's failure to have an erection is an indication that he is no longer attracted to her.

man's inability to have an erection is an indication of his lack of attraction to her. In most cases his attraction to his partner is certain, but a female partner's psyche is wired to assume that her man's arousal and erection is a direct expression of his attraction. He may not be able to persuade her that this is not true, no matter how attracted he is to her.

Partner reactions may be unsettling and extreme. How extreme may be determined by the history and quality of your relationship up until this point. In her pain and fear, your female partner may worry and fear the worst. If she tends towards being insecure, she may jump to the conclusion that your lack of excitement for her is evidence that you desire another woman or are being unfaithful. She may even express this in an accusatory fashion, making it difficult for you to avoid a defensive reaction. An extreme response by you may increase her worry about unfaithfulness rather than reassure her. If trust has been damaged in the history of your relationship, a failed erection can awaken her old wounds of hurt and distrust. From a prolonged pattern of sexual avoidance, her frustration may reach an extreme point of desperation in which she worries that you are gay and are not only not attracted to her, but not attracted to women in general. Again, the more extreme and defensive you are in your reaction to accusations, the greater the chance for a damaging moment while also increasing her worries about your sexual preference.

Painful moments have the potential to make your relationship much more complicated. Chaos is the result. Most couples have no script for sexual scenarios when their sexual play goes badly wrong. Female partners may feel upset by their partners' erection loss for extended periods of time. Multiple failed sexual experiences may cause her to feel anger, disappointment as well as insecure that her male partner is no longer attracted to her despite his assurances that it is not so. For her his limp penis is proof.

A woman may react with compassion by gently talking to her performance anxiety-afflicted man and telling him that she loves him, and all will be OK; hoping that her patience will solve the problem. Her patience, however, may diminish if his erection failures continue for a long duration, which oftentimes it does. Some women jump online to research the problem and attempt to convince their man that it is all in his head (which it is) and all he needs to do is relax (which is true), but his erection failures continue. Her patience transforms into frustration and hopelessness. Some women insist that their male partners get professional help (which they should), but for the man, his problems being the source of such acute shame and embarrassment, talking about them to a professional may be far too uncomfortable.

Other women become angry at being rejected, disappointed and found unattractive. For these women, the man's erection failure feels like an insult. She will attack, berate, criticize and belittle her man for his failures. Her insensitivities guarantee that his problems will continue and make the repair of his problem not only more difficult, but near impossible. A man who has been treated disrespectfully has a much greater difficulty regaining his confidence.

After the first failure, a female partner maybe willing in trying sex again to test if the problem persists, but after erection loss becomes a regular pattern, her appetite in exposing herself to more disappointment drops. She may develop contempt for her man who cannot "complete the job." Some female partners initially have a surge in sexual desire now that the male partner has discontinued initiating sex. But with repeated failures either in having sex or having successful sex, both partners become complicit in allowing their sex life to wither rather than face repeated failure, frustration, pain, and disappointment.

Emotional exercise 4: If you are in a relationship, learn from your sexual partner how she has been impacted by your performance anxiety. Let her express her all of her feelings about it. Her feelings may be difficult to hear. Request that this discussion to be non-judgmental and without criticism. Let it be an opportunity to learn about your partner; she is neither right nor wrong. Reassure her that you are determined in the course to solve this problem. Write down what your learn from her.

Sexual exercise 4: Redefine for yourself what a good enough erection is, based on your hardest recent erection instead of comparing it to when you were younger. Rate your hardest recent erection as a 10. Is it good enough for penetration? Write about this in your journal.

How Does Performance Anxiety Affect the Relationship?

The amount of unresolved pain contained between partners is directly related to the level of relationship satisfaction and health partners will experience. Already discussed is how when a man is stuck in the cycle of performance anxiety and cannot sexually succeed, both partners are in great pain. The pain will test their connection and at least strain it if not break it.

> Sex accounts is only a small percentage of a relationship, but once sex becomes a problem it infects 100% of the relationship.

Sex accounts for only a small percentage of time partners spend together within a love relationship. Once sex becomes a problem it infects all parts of the relationship. The entire relationship beyond sex may quickly become troubled, distorted, and awkward once sex ceases to function well. Activities that were easy and simple before erectile dysfunction became a problem become complicated because old behavior patterns no longer work well. Partners could previously relax with each other. Now, banter, sexual playfulness, affection, and teasing are no longer comfortable. Their absence leaves a void that has no substitute. Disappointment, pain, and anger are easily provoked.

The longer performance anxiety continues unsolved, the more partners intentionally create distance in their relationship because of the pain. They also stay away from the reality of lack of sexual connection. If too much time passes, the relevancy of the relationship falls away. The relationship becomes a zombie; a relationship in name only, without any real positive connection. Without solutions or improvements, the relationship is vulnerable to break-up.

Sexual exercise 5: Before beginning a sexual session, you and your partner will embrace unclothed for five full minutes. During your embrace, give intentional focus to the feeling of your partner's skin against yours. Take note of their heartbeat and feel it against you. Pay attention to their breathing and feel their inhales and exhales and how the rising and falling of his or her chest feels against you. Attempt to synchronize your breath with your partner's. Intentionally relax by letting go of everything other than what is in this moment. Include this practice each time before you intend to have sexual play. Record details of each experience in your journal.

Is the problem physical or emotional?

Men and their partners are uncertain about whether performance anxiety is a physically or emotionally based problem. When considering the specifics of the painful situation, some details of the difficulties seem to support both theories. An obvious conclusion is that the man is suffering from a physical problem because the issue is a lack of physical response, an erect penis. The belief that the man's body is broken in some way is consistent with what seems obvious.

Before seeking help from a sex therapist such as myself, Andrew Aaron, LICSW, many men and their partners first seek consultation with their physician, who routinely prescribes a pro-erection medicine such as Viagra, Cialis, or Levitra. At the request of the man and his partner, they will probably have a testosterone level test performed. As a sex therapist, my expertise is in the domain of emotions. I am able to offer those who seek my help are with their emotions. My unscientific estimate is that sex and sexual functioning are roughly 80% emotional. Though most people think of sex as a physical act, most far underestimate the huge role emotions play in sexual activity.

Upon use of the medicine, men may witness some limited success, once or twice before the problem of erection loss returns. The medicine can give a temporary boost from a "placebo effect," or the benefit that comes from the hope of improvement. Some men are provided with complete relief by the medicine if their hope of improvement is strong enough to lift them out of their emotionally based problem. Viagra and its pharmaceutical cousins are intended to help men with erection problems but are more effective at helping men who have erectile dysfunction caused by physical-based factors. In the situations of performance anxiety, the strength and power of a man's anxiety are far greater than the effectiveness of the medicine to improve blood flow to his penis. Emotions can be incredibly powerful, a fact usually significantly underestimated by most men.

Sometimes doctors prescribe testosterone supplements to men seeking help for performance anxiety, which may also provide temporary benefits, also due to a boost from a placebo effect. Poor or absent erections are also a symptom of low testosterone as well. The media has trained the male population, who are already insecure about their virility and sexual skills, that they all need more testosterone. Other symptoms of low testosterone are fatigue, low motivation, lack of or soft erections, lack of sexual desire, and sometimes depressive symptoms. Most men who work a lot and are suffering devastation from performance anxiety also feel fatigued, low motivation, lack of erections, lack of sexual desire, and depressive symptoms, so the condition of low testosterone may seem to be consistent. When the supplements don't solve the problem by restoring reliable erections, men and their doctors grow frustrated and hopeless enough that exploring the route of an emotionally-based cause becomes worth a try. It is all that is left. His doctor might then suggest that a therapist may help. However, a general therapist is not likely to have the necessary experience or expertise to be helpful. Performance anxiety is an emotional-based problem, but it is also mixed with sexual and relationship factors. However, men and their partners have suspected all along that the problem has been "all in his head."

> Performance Anxiety is an emotionally-based problem even though it shows up in physical ways, such as loss of erection.

Physically-based health conditions often contribute to erection problems. Health issues such as heart problems, circulatory problems, diabetes, high blood pressure, and/or obesity are associated with erection issues. The medicines used to treat these conditions are known to cause problems with erections as well. Most medicines are harmful to sexual functioning, sexual desire, arousal, and orgasm in both men and women, which will be discussed in greater detail later. Special consideration must be given to blood pressure medicine, which can prevent erections for many men. Anti-depressant medications are notorious for reducing sexual desire and for making orgasms difficult to achieve. However, some exceptional men do react to the anxiety-reduction offered by an anti-depressant with an exit from the cycle of performance anxiety, an easy solution to a complex problem. Some physicians prescribe medicine without warning patients of their sexual side effects. Physicians are not always aware of the negative sexual side effects of medications.

Possessing a psychological or emotional problem still carries a stigma that signifies weakness. If the source of erection loss was physical, a man may feel relieved that he may not be held personally responsible for the flaw. But if the problem is emotional then a man may worry that it is a personal weakness. Therefore, men prefer to stay away from the possibility of an emotional cause, up to the point of denial. Men also view a physical problem as easily defined and therefore more fixable. An emotionally-based problem that is all in his head is confusing, difficult to define, and feels out of control. Emotions reside within the realm of a "soft science," the gray areas instead of the world of black and white clarity. Men are more comfortable where all is clearly understood; where they can feel in control.

Emotional exercise 5: Think about your experience. Did you struggle in determining if your erection loss was physical or emotional? Are you certain right now about the source of your dysfunction?

Men and Their Emotions

Men, as a group, do not value their emotional selves. Men are socialized to value strength over sensitivity. A large distinction between females and males is that females, in the generally accepted characteristics of femininity, are allowed to show and express emotions. One way that men differentiate themselves from females is by disassociating themselves from their emotions to appear "tough and strong." Emotions suggest vulnerability to pain, the kind of weakness that men and their "Man Code" forbids. In the most masculine of activities and professions, men do not allow painful emotions to be expressed or to interfere with goal achievements, such as in construction, the military, or law enforcement. The man code dictates that men show only strength, which is limiting to men. Strength is not how much a man can lift; it is how much he can love.

> What men view as a "real man" often includes unrealistic ideals about masculinity.

The definition of masculinity has been refined by men and women for generations. Some qualities and attributes of men and masculinity have been developed through ideals, imagination, and myth. Femininity is also made up of distortions of who women really are. The concept of a "real man" is a collection of qualities, characteristics, ideals, and values that men use as a basis of comparison to determine if they are successful or good enough as men. What men view as a "real man" is often a collection of unrealistic ideals about masculinity.

If a man does not feel good about himself, he will look to the masculine ideal to determine where and how he must improve. Aspects of the masculine ideal are being strong, always in control, self-assured, always providing, and always capable. An expectation of the ideal is for a man to finish and succeed at tasks, with no possibility of failure, without feeling and with machine-like precision. Because of these beliefs, the opposites are also true; a man should never be afraid, be weak, out of control, or fail. Sexually, these ideals are true as well. A male sexual partner should always have an erection, be ready for sex, want sex all the time, and always be able to sexually satisfy his female partner. Of course, these standards are impossible and not human, but many men secretly use these principles as their guide. Unexpressed, they feel a failure when they don't measure up to these ideals. The unrealistic expectations a man has of himself contributes to how he reacts when his emotions begin to interfere with his sexual excitement and maintaining an erection during sex.

Confidence is a large factor in being masculine and in good sexual functioning. A male who does not feel confident will also not identify as masculine, as in the notion of being a "real man." Confidence and living up to the masculine ideal of the real man are the same. The widely held myth about masculinity is that a real man is always confident. This is an unhealthy standard because the true path to confidence is accepting our humanness, fears, and limitations, which can eventually lead to confidence. Sex is a challenging activity that is both natural and highly vulnerable at the same time. It is certain to provoke feelings of uncertainty and anxiety; feelings not associated with the myths of the real man.

Despite the internet and the prevalent availability of information, sexual knowledge is not received by everyone. Many people are not educated about sex and have limited, incorrect, or no information about sex. A man's lack of information erodes the very confidence he is supposed to have to be good enough. Not having enough information about a task in which success is highly important produces fear. A dilemma many sexually inexperienced young men find themselves in is that they feel the expectations of being in charge and the leader of sexual experiences while they simultaneously lack the necessary sexual information. Pressure is intensified by the rule forbidding the showing of vulnerability. The bind heightens anxiety because it is an impossible situation. For some men, the anxiety generated from this dilemma is the beginning of a permanent link between sex and anxiety. For some men, at the very beginning of their sexual career, they suffer erection loss that starts a lifelong pattern of sexual failure.

A large difference between men and their female counterparts is testosterone levels. Men's bodies generate and maintain much higher levels of the hormone. Among the influences of testosterone is a muted emotional experience. While men have the same feelings as women, men feel the emotions less strongly than women do, and more easily repress them, an act of burying them within. If feelings were heard as a voice, the volume of this voice would be much lower for men than for women. In the culture of men, this difference may account for valuing feelings less and dismissing them more. Despite testosterone, men have feelings but commonly disregard them.

Not considering their feelings much, men typically have little practice with emotional dynamics, an arena in which women are more aware and adept. Generally, women are more emotionally intelligent than men. They are more aware of their feelings, are skilled at putting words to them and expressing them. Women are more apt to be patient with their emotions and emotional process.

When it comes to men's feelings associated with vulnerability, such as fear, discomfort, anxiety, insecurity, inadequacy, and powerlessness, men tend to choose a singular one-size-fits-all reaction...repression. This practice contributes to the development of performance anxiety. Repression is the act of burying the feelings inside so that the pain is no longer felt. Repression effectively makes the feelings seem like they have gone away. They haven't gone away; the feelings are just buried so they are no longer a bother; they become unconscious. Repression is an emotional form of kicking the can down the road. It is also a way to strong-arm the feelings into submission with denial and rejection, not a good long-term choice from a mental health perspective. The alternative to repression is to feel the feelings and constructively channel them into action or words while accepting them, but men are often uncomfortable with the many feelings that represent vulnerability. They associate feelings with weakness.

Emotional exercise 6: Reflect on your definition of what is a "real man." Become more familiar with your behavior and choices to notice when the "man code" influences your words, actions, behaviors, and choices. Start paying close attention to the emotions that come and go throughout your days. Enter these in your journal.

Sexual exercise 6: Note in your journal about moments when thoughts of sex or daily situations resulted in having any kind of arousal that forms any slight, partial or full erection. Also note any presence of morning erection. A healthy man may wake up to an erection due to elevated levels of testosterone early in the morning. As men age this occurs less frequently. Some men wake to erections that seem to be related to the need to urinate.

Anxiety, Fear, Anger and Sex

Among the emotions that cause a man to feel weak is fear. A man violates the man code by admitting to fear or by looking afraid. To do so is a sign of weakness, which breaks the number one rule of masculinity. Fear and fear-based emotions such as worry, anxiety, nervousness, and panic are among the vulnerable emotions that many men seek to avoid. Performance anxiety, as the name indicates, is a form of anxiety. Most men who suffer from performance anxiety have lived with problematic anxiety much of their lives.

> Anxiety is an uncomfortable fear-based emotion that arises from worry or of feeling out of control.

Anxiety is an uncomfortable fear-based emotion that arises from worry or of feeling out of control. Fear and anxiety are powerful emotions that have a large role in performance anxiety. As an activity, sex may be successful and satisfying when there is no fear. Our bodies and our central nervous systems function well sexually when we are relaxed. A relaxed state is one in which we are safe from danger and threat. If danger and threat are present, our nervous systems are unavailable for sex because sexual activity will interfere with our ability to keep ourselves safe. In other words, if we are in danger, we should take action to ensure our safety; being sexual is not among these kinds of actions. Our bodies function to prioritize our survival over the need to connect with a partner, to have pleasure, or to reproduce.

A man's body and central nervous system express this reality by eliminating his ability for arousal and erection if he is afraid. A man may think of sex and desire sexual activity much of the time, but not if there is danger, a choice that could save his life. When threatened, we all experience what is called the "fight or flight response." We experience a neurologically heightened awareness and enhanced strength fueled by adrenaline to prepare to fight or run for our lives. A man who has an erection is unlikely to run or fight well! His life will be at risk. As a result, nature inhibits a man's ability to have an erection when he is afraid and threatened.

In the cycle of performance anxiety, the same dynamic is in force. Our nervous system does not make a distinction between the threat to his physical safety or the threat of failure. A man who worries about disappointing himself or his female partner feels under threat; because of it, he loses his erection. For the man, the situation of failure is dangerous to his well-being and survival as a "good-enough" man.

Anxiety is a fear-based emotion that ranges in intensity from mild to severe. In our fast-paced society, anxiety is at epidemic proportions. Stress plays a significant role in the development of anxiety difficulties. Its high prevalence in no way diminishes the discomfort and debilitating effect anxiety may have.

At the mild end of the spectrum, anxiety is an annoying discomfort, such as being on edge with a mild inability to relax. When more severe, anxiety can disable a person from functioning and living a normal life. Panic is a brief but intensely negative experience that shows up as an attack or acute episode. A large panic attack is most severe; it can seem like a heart attack in which the sufferer feels like he or she is going crazy or dying. Those who survive a large panic attack routinely go to the emergency department fearing a heart attack.

In families where parents have anxiety-based conditions, the behavior patterns, thought processes, and values associated with anxiety contribute to impressing an anxiety-based perspective upon their children. In this way, rather than an inherited genetic condition, though a propensity for anxiety may exist, parents and families teach their children to have anxiety and model it by example.

Worrying is a thought process and a cognitive habit that is present in anxiety disorders. Worry is a non-productive, negative thought pattern that is a future-oriented focus on bad, negative, hurtful, and even catastrophic potential future events. Parents who have anxiety may express to their children countless times to "be careful" or "watch out for bad people." Such statements repeatedly warn of dangers and contribute to anxiety "training." Worrying is part of an unhealthy anxious pattern not just because it inflates the size or likelihood of potential future dangers, but it tends to disable the worrier in anticipation of dangerous developments rather than truly establishing effective preparation to minimize for such occurrences.

A link exists between angry feelings and the development of anxious reactions. When angry feelings are habitually repressed instead of constructively expressed, they get indirectly channeled into anxiety. As a result, should an anger-provoking incident occur, anxiety may be triggered and linger at a high level for some time afterward.

Avoidance is a behavior pattern of those who are anxious as a way of keeping the level of anxiety low. It is a negative pattern that is limiting in nature. Avoidance has the high cost of reducing the quality of life. To avoid unpleasant or threatening situations, some attempt to assert control over others or situations which produces secondary negative results that harm relationships and discourages growth.

Anxiety shows up in people's lives in many forms, such as Generalized Anxiety Disorder, Obsessive/Compulsive Disorder (OCD), Panic Disorder, Post-traumatic Stress Disorder (PTSD), phobias, health anxiety, perfectionism, jealousy, and insecurity. In each of these disorders,

> Anxiety and sex are not friends.

anxiety is present with differing behaviors and differing intensities. At a high intensity, each disorder makes the quality of life poor and daily functioning difficult and perhaps impossible, including sexual functioning. Men who become troubled with performance anxiety usually have lived with forms of problematic anxiety long before the development of erectile dysfunction and sexually-based difficulties. Their anxiety made them susceptible to it.

Anxiety is detrimental to good sex. The quality of a sexual experience is directly related to the level of partner relaxation: the more relaxed means better sex. When anxious, partners are less self aware, less available for connection, less able to become aroused, maintain arousal, and less able to achieve orgasm. An anxious partner is less present to participate in a satisfying sexual experience. One who has experienced trauma may also be sexually inhibited or so withdrawn that they do not sexually "show up," by becoming aroused, participating in reciprocal pleasuring or experience sex as a pleasurable activity.

Men who suffer from general anxiety are more vulnerable to performance anxiety than men who are not challenged with it. A man who develops performance anxiety has probably experienced episodes of distressing anxiety in a variety of forms, such as general anxiousness, panic attacks, or old unresolved trauma. These men practice avoidance of feelings that tend to increase anxiety. Men whose functioning is not limited by anxiety are less likely to get caught in the performance anxiety trap because they react by challenging the anxiety to calm themselves.

Performance anxiety is an anxiety disorder. Men who suffer from it will need to develop greater emotional strength to calm and soothe all their difficult emotions, but especially their anxiety. To overcome this sexually-based dysfunction, a man must become better at coping with anxiety-provoking life situations, including those that have nothing to do with sex.

A source of anxiety for both men and women is the challenge of anger. Daily life is complicated and stressful. A normal day in our lives includes moments of anger, the emotion we have when a situation is not to our liking. When we are hurt or blocked, we experience of anger; energy mobilized to resist or oppose the experience. Anger is a broad spectrum of emotions that range from low to high intensity. Annoyance is a low-intensity angry feeling whereas being enraged is a high-intensity angry feeling. Other angry feelings are irritation, frustration, fuming, being heated, being upset, being mad and being pissed. Angry feelings are normal but are not useful unless the energy is directed towards positive action.

The connection between anger and depression is strong and direct. Depression is usually caused by a maladaptive use of anger and the substantial energy contained within it. The energy mobilized in anger has a purpose: to fix, eliminate or remove the problematic issue. The angry energy and action are a solid team. When the team is split up, we are less well. When that energy is habitually internalized instead of used for a purpose, depression results. Solving problems is best and is a great way to be kind to yourself. If we regularly fix problems with the energy when anger has been provoked, we prevent depression. All too often, we do not have the power or control to influence an issue, such as when a boss acts insensitively, an economy is unfavorable, or a romantic partner behaves inconsiderately. Repressing anger when we have no power or control will shut us down into depression, an emotional state in which we disappear to ourselves. In depression we emotionally become disconnected from our own personal power. At its worst, depression can be dangerous to our survival. When lost in a deep depressive episode, we have the feeling of powerlessness.

A strong link exists between anger and personal power. Power is the ability to love and make our lives the way we want them to be. A widely accepted misunderstanding is that power is used for force. Rarely is force constructive; while it may achieve the desired results, it may do so while causing collateral damage. Anger is a closed emotion with opposition or resistance to an undesirable situation. Anger alone does not include addressing the problem, fixing it, or creating a solution. Openness is required to create solutions. Fixing problems and creating solutions makes our lives and love relationships better...that is REAL power.

In the masculine world, power, force, and strength are common to most male activities, for instance, competition is a drama of proving who has the most power. As a result, men see themselves and the

> For men, our penises are our original "power tool."

world through a perspective of power. A man who is unable to perform sexually experiences significant powerlessness, an experience that may seem to him as non-masculine. Love is accomplished by letting go of power and being open. Force is rarely helpful to love, with the exception of certain kinds of partner-accepted moments of playfulness. The kind of power men identify with as masculine includes the power to sexually succeed. The old word for erection loss is "impotence," which is a word that also means powerless.

For men, our penises strongly represent our power. An erection is symbolic of our masculine power. Construction is widely seen as a manly activity in which power tools are used. For men, our penises are our original "power tool." Erection loss is associated with feelings of powerlessness. Anger is also associated with power; but only if we succeed at using the energy from anger to create a good outcome. If accomplished regularly, life will get better and better as anger-provoking problems are solved. But men who get trapped in the cycle of performance anxiety do not use their anger effectively. Instead, they internalize their anger due to feeling powerless and to avoid conflict. Internalizing is the act of burying the feeling within instead of expressing it in words or actions. Expressing it is powerful whereas internalizing is a choice that detrimentally separates the energy from power.

Most often anger comes in many small doses. Moments of frustration, irritability, and annoyance are much more common than moments when we are greatly angered. Habitually internalizing these small doses of anger causes men to feel more and more powerless. The experience of powerlessness is increasing for most of us in our society as corporations grow larger, forces around us are less sensitive to our well-being, and the internet shields many systems from accountability and responsiveness. Being powerful in our lives does not have to come from changing the world, but the ability to adjust ourselves so the world and daily developments do not unsettle us. We have a choice about our inner state.

A man who is caught in the trap of performance anxiety has surrendered his power and no longer has control of his inner balance. Continuously internalizing anger erodes a man's balance, the power to achieve it, and to maintain it. As anger gets stuffed within, it builds, and the angry energy surfaces as anxiety or anxiety disorders.

If a man is able to face a difficult situation and channel his energy away from anger and instead into the constructive action of fixing or resolving the problem, he will become increasingly powerful in creating a satisfying life, love relationship, and sexual play. If the energy is not blocked by holding onto and internalizing anger, the energy will flow in his life. Flowing energy feels alive. Blocked energy causes us to get stuck and contributes to powerlessness and dysfunction.

Emotional exercise 7: Write in your journal about how you experience anxiety, anger, depression, and power. At the end of each day, write down instances of anxiety and how you calmed it or reacted to it. Recall and record events that caused you to feel angry. Also make note of situations in which you feel powerless. Write down what you felt in reaction to being powerless and what you did with these feelings.

Sexual exercise 7: Continue to get together often with your partner for non-intercourse sexual play. Excluding intercourse can be difficult and even frustrating, especially for some female partners. Talk about this together. Absolutely stay away from intercourse. One sexual disappointment can eliminate the benefits of all your actions. Continue to learn of and discover new and varied ways to give and receive sexual pleasure. Have the two of you tried anything new which may become a favorite? Slow sex way down.

Include slow, sensuous massage. While you do so, both of you should relax deeply while paying attention to your breathing. Give each other slow full-body massages after the long embrace and before beginning sexual play in each intimate session.

The Relationship with Your Penis

How a man views himself directly determines the quality of his masculinity. For both men and women, the level of self-esteem or relationship with oneself strongly influences the perspective of one's body as poor, good enough, or satisfying. Women with low self-esteem often express inner self-dislike by seeing their bodies as unattractive and undesirable. A similar dynamic is true for men regarding their penises, a man's singular greatest expression of masculinity. The relationship a man has with his penis is special with no real female counterpart. The closest female equivalent are breasts. A man who suffers from very low self-esteem is vulnerable to feeling that his penis is insufficient. For men, penis size is a big deal (pun intended). In a man's psyche, the larger his penis the more masculine he is. If a man feels bad about himself, it may be true that no matter how large his penis is, he will feel that it is not big enough. This joke shares a basic truth: "Breasts come in two sizes: too large and too small, but penises come in only one size: too small!"

Contrary to the traditional belief that a dog is a man's best friend, closer to the truth is that a man's penis is his best friend. Men experience their penis as a separate entity, having a mind all its own. There is a ring of truth when women say that "he was thinking with his other head." Men notice, sometimes with horror, that their penises react independently and inconsistently to the intent of their owner. This is especially true when a young man's penis becomes erect at inconvenient and embarrassing moments. For more mature men suffering from performance anxiety, the opposite is unfortunately true; their penises do not respond when an erection is desired. Many men view their penis as an add-on piece of equipment that is separate from his person with a separate will. It seems so distinct that some men have given their penises affectionate names as would a separate individual.

Men also look to their penises with friendly affection regarding pleasure and self-soothing. Most men enjoy touching and fondling it and enjoy being touched by their partners as well. To do so is relaxing. The friendship between a man and his penis extends to the pleasure he feels from masturbation. It is a way men choose to have pleasure, while also calming themselves when anxious, stressed, worried, or doubtful. If very anxious, some men are prone to masturbate compulsively, a never-ending cycle in reaction to inner anxiety and low self-esteem. Frequent masturbation is not a problem unless it causes soreness, interferes with fulfilling daily responsibilities, or interferes with the good quality of a relationship. A man's first sexual responsibility is to fulfill his female partner's satisfaction before satisfying himself through masturbation.

As men age, so do their penises. Aging affects the penis and sexual functioning significantly. Though if a man remains physically healthy, he should be able to have a good enough erection for intercourse into his old age. Most medications negatively affect sexual functioning, desire, arousal, erection, and ejaculation. The negative influences of medicine increase with aging and the coincidental health complications. Beware of blood pressure medications; a common side effect is reduced or impaired erections.

As men age, their erections are not as hard, penises become erect more slowly, penises need more direct stimulation to stay hard and may experience ejaculation and orgasm as less intense than when they were younger. As we age, we become more sensitive to every negative influence. Factors which had no before impact gradually begin to. Emotions, distractions, stress, health problems, unresolved relationship problems all interfere as never before. Aging happens so slowly that men often do not initially notice any change.

Erections are the result of blood flow to the penis. A man's overall health, his heart and vascular system get reflected in a man's erection. Without a strong heart and vascular system that can maintain sufficient blood flow and pressure, an erection would not be possible. Your general health determines and supports your erections. Maintaining your health with a good diet, regular exercise while remaining fit is the way to protect healthy sexual functioning. As your health goes, so does your erection.

The effects of aging can cause a man to fall into the trap of performance anxiety. Men don't always notice the very gradual effects of aging on their penises and on sexual response. So in moments when they suddenly awaken to the age-related changes about which they have been unaware, men become upset and believe something is wrong. In actuality, their awareness has caught up to their aging. The upset and subsequent anxiety can result in a cycle of performance anxiety that is difficult to reverse.

Sexual Desire

Most men experience significant sexual desire. Virility, or the quality of masculinity, is also a feature of what most expect from a "real man." Strong and incessant sexual desire are considered masculine attributes. However, there are myths of masculinity that deviate from how most men truly are. Men individually and collectively experience a range of amount and intensity of sexual desire. Younger men tend to feel more high sexual desire than do older men, though there are always exceptions. Men feel sexual desire as a physically-located urging and need. Some men feel sexual desire so strongly that it does not feel optional; they experience of sexual desire as a need. Each man, however, has the responsibility to cope with desire, and must be curbed at appropriate times to protect himself and others.

Within the ranks of men are also those who do not have much desire for sex. Because of how a "real man" is defined and myths about masculinity, men with low sexual desire are not likely to acknowledge or announce it. Their low level of sexual interest can be a point of shame. Men come in all intensities of sexual desire from low to high, but the masculine myths only recognizes those at the high end as truly being masculine.

Subscribing to the masculine myth, female partners of men with lower sexual desire feel disappointed and frustrated that their man is not manly. Female partners who are the main sexual initiators in their relationships miss feeling desired and the experience of an assertive male partner pursuing them. The discrepancy of desire, when partners have different levels of sexual desire, can cause tension, conflict, and pain between partners if unresolved. Most partners feel disappointed when their partner desires sex more or less frequently than them. Female partners of men who have high desire also complain that their men want sex too much. Men with high and incessant desire, those wanting sex daily or more, sometimes get labeled by their partners pathologically as sex addicts. No matter what the specific source of a problem, negativity and uncomfortable emotions may fuel the cycle of performance anxiety.

Men who have suffered past trauma, especially childhood sexual abuse, may not possess much sexual desire and they may actively avoid sex. Yet many men do experience chronic, intense, and incessant sexual desire. As a group, men do not complain much about this reproductive burden, yet privately the persistent sexual cravings can be frustrating, nagging, distracting, and inconvenient. Men suffer from sexual desire and it causes problems. If a man were to drive a muscle car for the first time, without skill or experience at driving such a powerful car, he may crash. Without emotional balance and inner strength, men struggle to control the power of their sex drive. Some do crash by sexually acting out.

An aspect of strength and being a "real man" paradoxically also includes the strength to control his sexual desire so that he is always a responsible, non-hurtful individual. A great car may be powerful, but even the most powerful car is only good if it has effective brakes. This balance for some men is difficult to achieve.

What is a normal level of sexual desire? Normal or healthy represents a wide range. A man who desires sex daily is equally within the normal range as a man who is satisfied with sex twice a month. What is normal and healthy is determined more by how his sexual desire is expressed and ways he chooses to satisfy his desire. If his sexual needs are expressed in negative ways, through risky behaviors that negatively impact his partner or in ways that cause shame, then he may be increasing the fuel for being trapped in the cycle of performance anxiety.

Emotional exercise 8: Reflect on your definition of what a "real man" is. Make a list of the qualities you believe make up a "real man." Have you tried to develop some of these qualities? Have you felt badly about yourself because you believe you lack these qualities? What qualities can you develop so you can be proud of yourself? Write these answers down.

Sexual exercise 8: During sexual play, include times when you manually pleasure your penis to erection. Incorporate times when your partner manually and orally pleasures your penis, so long as it can be done without discomfort for either of you. If you succeed in achieving an erection, both of you express admire for the erection and express love for your penis. Include this exercise in some of your future sexual sessions.

The Health of Emotions

As mentioned previously, the relationship between men and their emotions is not a positive one. This is especially true with uncomfortable feelings. For men emotions are an inconvenience that they would do away with if they could, and most try to. Unlike women who experience a broad spectrum of emotions, men identify experiencing just a few emotions. The emotional muting due to high levels of testosterone is one cause, masculine socialization that rejects emotion is another, but men will habitually repress their negative emotions because to feel them is to give those feelings the potential to interfere with the success of goals. They may also interfere with his appearance as strong.

Men just have a few feelings they identify. A point of masculine pride for men is derived from not allowing painful feelings to prevent them from achieving their goals. The first major feeling that men identify is "Everything is OK." Men experience this emotion when their world is generally in order. The second one is anger, which may be the only actual emotion they acknowledge feeling. Men can be good at getting angry. Because power is a significant component of masculinity, large and loud anger feels powerful to men and therefore they do not identify it as problematic. But, a major problem plaguing many men is of anger being demonstrated too powerfully and causing damage or hurt. Men must control impulses so that they never use more force in anger than is required to solve a problem. Men's last identifiable feeling is a combination of hungry/horny/tired and a desire to watch a sporting event. The horny feeling is absent from men who fear erection failure due to performance anxiety. As simple as it seems, this is emotional repertoire of most men.

His negative relationship with his feelings makes him vulnerable to performance anxiety. Knowing and managing his feelings well is necessary to succeed in all phases of life including sex. Men who tend to reject feelings by burying them, fail to develop emotional awareness, and are often unable to express feelings with words or soothe uncomfortable feelings to reduce them. This sets men up for the trap of performance anxiety.

When a man first experiences erection loss, he may react with horror, fear, worry, and emotionally shut down to reject his pain. Or in a superior way, if he is emotionally aware and strong, he may remain open to his partner while calming his uncomfortable emotions. If he is successful, he and his partner may return to loving and pleasuring each other in ways that do not require an erection. By shifting his focus away from negative feelings instead of becoming alarmed, a repair, which may include an erection, may be possible later. When we have a painful problem, we may make it bigger by responding in a negative and ineffective way. We can make the problem smaller by reacting in a positive and strong way. When confronted with an uncomfortable situation, we may invest our energy in the negative emotions, which inflates them, or withdraw our energy from those same negative emotions and reduce them.

By possessing emotional intelligence and awareness, men are empowered to calm and soothe their uncomfortable feelings, an effort that makes painful problems smaller. When repressing or rejecting difficult feelings such as fear, anxiety and anger, men lose the ability to calm themselves. They also lose the ability to maintain their balance, which is absolutely necessary for continued arousal and erection.

The term emotional intelligence refers to self-awareness, emotional awareness, and the competency at identifying feelings. Emotional intelligence includes the strength of working with feelings, expressing them, and understanding others' feelings. Emotional intelligence also includes the ability to act towards others with the compassion gained from understanding how they feel, especially valuable partners in a love relationship. Because of the tendency to mute and repress their emotions, men as a group are less emotionally intelligent than women who are not restricted by the "man code." Being stuck in the trap of performance anxiety is evidence that a man needs to develop increased emotional intelligence.

Love relationships are emotional entities. A connection between partners is

> Stuck in the trap of performance anxiety is evidence that a man needs to develop increased emotional intelligence.

built through the sharing of emotions and emotional experiences. Understanding a partner's emotional experience strengthens the bonds of connection. Acting and reacting with sensitivity and compassion, especially to painful feelings, make a connection stronger. Reflecting back a partner's emotions, such as reacting with joy when a partner has a success, makes the connection between partners stronger while also allowing a partner to feel understood. Not only will greater awareness help restore the ability to have an erection during sex, but also provides each man with access to a better-quality love relationship and connection.

Emotional exercise 9: Reflect on the emotions you experience. Identify some of the emotions you have recently felt. Are there any emotions you feel more frequently than any others? Name and list them in your journal.

The Emotional Nature of Sex

Sex is a dynamic exchange between sexual partners. Most female partners prize an emotional connection as among the most important elements of good sex. Great sex is possible when both partners are most alive and highly aroused. And in great sex, little is more of a turn-on than a totally excited partner. As will be discussed more later, the quality of the relationship between sexual partners is a huge factor in a man's arousal and the quality of his erection.

Good sex can be imagined as an upward spiral, in which each partner adds some excitement that fuels the other's excitement in a back-and-forth upward exchange. Round and round, the couple is lifted up in pleasure and connection. The foundation of great sex is built from partners offering openness and connection. At its best, the partners lift each other up in pleasure and excitement to an intensely high level.

Sex is holistic. This means that all the influences of daily experiences, emotions, and issues, like stresses and strains, do not stop at the threshold of the bedroom door when partners are sexual. Negative life factors can dampen the excitement if partners don't have the emotional strength to put them to the side. Partner tension, resentments and distrust all may cause partners to maintain walls of defensiveness. Cautious, untrusting partners are partially closed. Negative emotions cause partners to be closed which reduces pleasure and connection. Complete openness maximizes the potential for great sex. The emotional nature of sex means that the most positive emotions act as fertilizer in the garden of pleasure. Some of the emotions that encourage openness and safety are love, admiration, gratitude, kindness, and desire.

Performance Anxiety: A Self-fulfilling Prophecy

The dynamics of performance anxiety are simple. A man is trapped in a bind. He feels a lot of pressure from within to sexually succeed. He may experience this pressure from his female partner as well. Male partners wish to avoid disappointing her and dread instances of her upset. A man who has experienced erection loss or failure is terrified of repeating this. Moments of sexual failure are among the worst moments a man can have. Men may actively avoid sex if not confident of success, but a persistent female partner can only be put off for so long. The fear a man feels about erection loss causes his fight or flight reaction to become active. In his fear, he repeatedly worries about the specifics of the breakdown, the embarrassment, the inadequacy, and his upset female partner. As he worries, his anxiety increases, as does the intensity of his fight or flight response. Being preoccupied with fear results in the man's attention being focused on his thoughts in his head instead of focused on his body where his attention needs to be for good sex. He experiences a lack of physical sensation which is blocked by his fear which further alienates him from his arousal. His fear of losing his erection becomes a certainty as he once again has erection failure and loss. This cycle repeats each time a sexual experience is anticipated. As the self-fulfilling prophecy is energized, he fears that he will fail, which guarantees that he will.

Some men find reprieve from this cycle when a sexual experience is initiated spontaneously without any planning or preparation. Spontaneous sex interrupts the performance anxiety cycle by taking away the male partner's anticipatory worry about failure and poor performance. A spontaneous encounter initiated by his female partner literally does not provide him the time to think about failure. A good performance with a solid erection can occur this way. Some couples saddled with performance anxiety create a new style of sex from this discovery of success where the female partner initiates sex without warning. It may work, but usually only for limited periods of time. A solid solution that comes from growth and healing is more satisfying for both partners and allows for more fluid and frequent sexual opportunities. The ultimate solution is superior because it includes male partner strengthening and growth.

Emotional exercise 10: Write in your journal how your experience of performance anxiety forms a self-fulfilling prophecy. Have you ever made attempts to avoid sex after first experiencing erection loss? Specifically note the anticipatory fear you have felt prior to sex. Have you had the experience yet of calming your fear/anxiety and then had sexual success?

For the Single Man

Some men who have become trapped in the grip of performance anxiety do not have a romantic partner. Single men find themselves in a very uncomfortable spot. Lacking the confidence that comes with the ability to maintain an erection, many men avoid dating. Being single results in a very uncomfortable bind; they don't have the sexual confidence to risk a new relationship, but will require a relationship and a partner for an active sex life to recapture his confidence.

A single man has the freedom and privacy to practice masturbation. Men without partners know acutely the difference between the level of anxiety of solo sex versus partner sex. They painfully know of anxiety's impact on erections. The fear that is generated by a romantic opportunity quickly distorts a man's perception of the priority that a potential female partner places on sex. Most women value sex, but do not believe that a first date needs to be or ought to be sexual. Because men place a high value on their penis and sex that they often incorrectly assume that female partners do the same. Many men who are insecure about their erections, fear that a new potential romantic partner will expect sex right away and will reject him when he fails to pass the sexual satisfaction test. A more confident man does not rush sex because he has nothing to prove. He will allow a relationship to develop gradually and will sense when his woman has sexual interest instead of anxiously seeking to prove his capabilities.

Unlike men in relationships, single men do not get to practice tolerating the stress of a real sexual scenario. Athletes gain much improvement in skill from practice, but no amount of practice equals real game experience. That is the disadvantage a single man has when he wishes to overcome the erectile dysfunction of performance anxiety.

Don't hold back from seeking a partner. A dating scenario offers an erection-troubled man powerful opportunities to grow. To meet with a potential partner when a man lacks confidence demands that he faces his fear. But if the courage to face his fear only results in painful disappointments the cycle of performance anxiety will grip more tightly instead of loosening. Be willing to start a new relationship based on being real and open. You will find that honesty and openness is refreshing and valuable.

A route is of humility, openness and honesty. When a single man is willing to accept that his value is not just based upon his ability to sexually perform he will find hope. He is more than just his penis. As will be explored later, when a man starts to value himself and discontinue hiding behind his shame, he has an opportunity to climb out the painful pit into which he has fallen.

Being real with a new potential partner through openness and honesty gives a man the possibility of increase in strength. As will be explored later, being able to calm his anxiety and self-negating attitude are steps towards overcoming the debilitating erection loss by evaluating himself and his emotions. Determining moments that are safe and unsafe to participate in intercourse instead of setting himself up for failure can help to earn admiration from a new potential partner. These strategies are discussed in the future chapters but are discussed within the context of a man who is in a relationship. The dynamics will be the same for the single man as he establishes a new relationship.

The Solution: A Team Effort

When in the grips of performance anxiety, the way out of the problem can seem complex and impossible. The solution is simple, though challenging. On the surface, it is a one-partner problem. If only the male partner could reliably have an erection, all the fuss and drama could go away. However, if that male partner is part of a couple, to create a lasting solution, we must create a two-partner repair.

A positive emotional environment supports arousal and good sex. Having worked with many men who are stuck in the cycle of performance anxiety and the couples whose relationships are strained by it, time and again it is proven that the solution has to be gradually put in place while the couple remains actively sexual. Otherwise, tensions build and the lack of a positive environment interferes with the achievement of success. This can be compared to a highway that needs resurfacing while traffic continues to flow on it. A positive environment includes the following ingredients: a relaxed state between both partners, hopefulness, sexual experiences that are stress and pressure-free, and partners who feel well-connected. With these favorable conditions, the environment is optimal for the male partner to be able to maintain his arousal and erection.

A solution also must include a male partner who has become better at calming his anxious feelings by developing greater emotional awareness. He has to have skillfully developed the ability to work with his difficult emotions in order to protect his inner balance. His mind will have to remain calmer, while he uses his strength effectively to soothe inner turmoil so it can stay at a minimum and protect his arousal.

The solution includes a man who understands the conditions in which he can and cannot sexually succeed. He creates for himself and his partner a more comfortable relationship situation in which respect is maintained and negativity is reduced. Another way that a man succeeds at loosening the grip of performance anxiety is by determining when the conditions are poor, such as when he is stressed, tired, preoccupied, or is disconnected from his romantic partner, judiciously using his strength to say "no" to intercourse. In this way he builds

> A man makes himself proud when he knows his limitations and sets himself up for success.

confidence when he makes promises and fulfills them but knows when to not make a promise because he cannot fulfill it. A man makes himself proud when he knows his limitations and sets himself up for success under both favorable and unfavorable conditions.

Perfection is never expected. Partners must be able to handle real-life circumstances with the strength to cope. The solutions we aim to create do not assume that success will be achieved during every sexual experience. Unlike the unrealistic masculine ideal, real circumstances and real men and women produce human results, not perfect results. As couples work to escape the vicious cycle of performance anxiety, failures will undoubtedly happen. Resilience is required so that after a setback, a man may regroup and be ready to succeed in the next sexual opportunity. As male partners grow in confidence, the possibility of repair during sex is a valuable and important skill. To be able to cope with failures, disappointments, difficulties, and unexpected results, a man must be able to calm himself and re-orient his focus in a new direction. He can reconnect with his partner with renewed intention and put that which didn't work behind him with a new life lesson and a possibility of a regained erection once he is rebalanced. Not all goes according to plan. Being adjustable, flexible, and adaptable are strengths that benefit every man and every couple.

A final part of the solution is the inclusion of a supportive, patient and positive female partner. Most women in a couple strained by performance anxiety also have great discomfort. Her pain comes into the sexual arena as much as his does. In her disappointment and frustration, if she is not part of the team to achieve a solution, her emotions and attitude have the potential to undermine her man's success. In instances where her unhappiness and disappointment unsettles her male partner's arousal, all the efforts for success are diminished, and eventually come to nothing.

Building solutions is an act of balancing forces. Partners will have to be strong enough to maintain a finely tuned sense of stability. If partners do not have sufficient impulse control, a moment of distress can very quickly destroy any progress that has been made.

Early on in this course, intercourse was discontinued. The purpose of doing so was to reduce the pressure and pain caused by the sexual dysfunction. The foundation of a positive environment upon which solutions can be built is vital. Once this foundation is established and becomes more solid, intercourse may be re-introduced when the risk of relapse is low.

Emotional exercise 11: Reflect on the dynamics between you and your partner. Identify experiences where you and your painful feelings and your partner's feelings contributed to a disappointing experience. Are there any experiences when either you or your partner successfully coped with difficult feelings so that the sexual experience rebounded to success? Write your answers in the journal.

Emotional exercise 12: While using the relaxation exercise, when the audio is ended, focus your attention on your pelvis, penis and testicles for 5 minutes. Be very detailed by scanning small areas the size of a dime; one spot after the next with your attention. Allow your attention to rest on each part 10-15 seconds as you feel the sensations in each location. Imagine warmth, your love, energy and blood flowing to these parts. As you do this, imagine these body parts becoming stronger and healthier. Include this at the end of every instance of using the relaxation exercise moving forward.

Maintaining Arousal

Sex is natural. When sex goes well, it is easy and simple; the way it should be. But when sex is troubled, it becomes highly complicated. Simplifying it can seem like an impossible task. An effort that helps by both partners is becoming more relaxed.

Relaxation is a state of being that allows for optimum arousal and provides the best possible conditions for the best sex and male performance. Being relaxed is simple in concept. However, a sexual situation is a demanding environment. A sexual situation is as vulnerable as situations can be. During sex, we must balance extreme closeness, nakedness and expectation with complete vulnerability. These truths underlie a reason why performance anxiety develops in the sexual arena.

We live in a busy, pressure-filled, complex world that does not support being relaxed. Yet our health is maintained by returning to a relaxed state as much as possible. During time off from our jobs, we often engage in some form of recreation, which literally means "re-creation," when we RE-create ourselves. The activities we choose to recreate almost always include some form of relaxation. It is by relaxing that we reset ourselves and return to balance after being imbalanced by everyday pressures and stressors.

By engaging regularly in deliberate relaxation exercises, you will be rebalancing your health and yourself. You will also start to build a supportive environment where you can maintain your arousal and your erection during sex. As you consciously practice to relax, try to be aware of your level of anxiety throughout each day. Also, practice calming and reducing your level of anxiety intentionally from time to time every day. This can be done by letting go of torment or worry. This practice will bear fruit during future sexual experiences when relaxing yourself will help you maintain your erection. Being aware of internally-held anxiety or stress gives you the chance to let it go. Up until now, you have probably been unaware of it and therefore unable to let it go.

Relaxing is the first step towards a shift in how you know yourself. The shift is from knowing yourself through external factors to learning about yourself from what you find within. Confidence is key for your sexual success. It comes from an improved quality of relationship with yourself. As you look within, you will grow increasingly familiar with your real self, made not from your thinking, but from your feeling, and

> Confidence is key for your sexual success. It comes from an improved quality of relationship with yourself.

awareness of your inner experience. Knowing yourself comes with the benefit of greater emotional stability because your deeper inner world fluctuates less than the outer world. If who you are is based on external events, then you feel valuable when you have a good day and worthless if you have a bad day. Imagine only being valuable if the sun is shining? Variations like this make you unstable and prone to suffering.

Emotional exercise 13: Have you experienced moments when you were relaxed and succeeded in having and maintaining an erection (this could be when alone or with your partner)? Have you noticed a connection between your level of anxiety, your level of relaxation and the quality and duration of your erections?

Sexual exercise 9: Time to re-evaluate your sexual play. Talk with your partner about the conditions of your emotional connection with her. If your erection has been reliable during recent partner sex and you have felt confident, consider trying a short duration (30 seconds) of intercourse. Keep the duration short. Keep your expectations low. Allow this to be an experience of intercourse without vigorous thrusting and without it leading to orgasm for either of you. Gentle and slow instead. Stay away from pressuring yourself for large success. Avoid a prolonged visit inside your partner. If this is a positive experience without anxiety or pressure, include short durations of intercourse in your sexual sessions moving forward, if the conditions support success. If you experience loss of erection, then discontinue intercourse and shift to other forms of sexual pleasuring.

Identifying and Naming Your Feelings

You experience a broad spectrum of emotions every day. Becoming aware of these feelings will open your life to a richer daily experience. Being more aware of your feelings has the potential to give you access to your personal power, greater balance, greater resiliency, improved connection in your love relationship, and success at escaping the trap of performance anxiety.

EMOTIONS

Tuning in to your emotions requires greater sensitivity. Men have generally rejected sensitivity; the man code has taught them that sensitivity is for women. That belief has dulled you. The attitude many men have suggests that they view sensitivity as weakness. Once you understand that strength and sensitivity go hand in hand, a door will open to allow growth. For instance, an eagle's eye is so sensitive that it can see prey from a mile above. A great NFL wide-receiver is so sensitive to his quarterback's timing that he is prepared to successfully receive a pass at forty yards. Similarly, by being sensitive to your own feelings, you may create successes in your life that were previously inaccessible.

Here are some emotions with which you may already be familiar. This is a short incomplete list. Many other emotions that people feel are not on this list. Get familiar with these feelings:

Happy	Sad	Joy	Angry
Relaxed	Disappointed	Thrilled	Frustrated
Peaceful	Unhappy	Excited	Irritated
Content	Insecure	Amazed	Annoyed
Fulfilled	Worried	Eager	Agitated
Satisfied	Jealous	Elated	Mad
Pleased	Afraid	Gleeful	Upset
Proud	Nervous	Ecstatic	Heated

Emotions fall along a spectrum from comfortable to uncomfortable. Our feelings are all equally part of our human experience. While some feel good and others feel bad, they are all equally an expression of you. If we can accept all feelings as equally worthy instead of valuing them by their level of comfort, the possibilities in our lives increase dramatically.

> While some emotions feel good and others feel bad, they are all equally an expression of your self.

Tolerating uncomfortable feelings is difficult but tolerating a poor quality of life and the problem of performance anxiety is worse! Performance anxiety is the result of being selective in which feelings you accept and reject.

Our challenge is to live with the painful feelings. The ones that feel good are rarely a problem. To address your area of weakness, pay special attention to the uncomfortable feelings in the list. Become more familiar with these. They represent painful and difficult situations in your life. It is normal to react to undesirable events with anger and fear. Notice them more. Puts words to your feelings. Allow yourself to feel them without pushing them away or burying them. They will be uncomfortable and you can tolerate them. Check in with your feelings regularly through your days by feeling them. Notice if they stay the same or if they change. Pay attention to their intensity and quality. If your feelings were a song, the intensity is like the volume and the kind of feeling is like the melody.

FEAR AND ANXIETY

Become an expert regarding your fear-based and anger-based feelings. By failing to get erect, your penis has been telling you that too much of your power has been tied up in fear and anger. Fear-based feelings include being afraid, anxious, worried, jealous, insecure, and suspicious. These are very common feelings. The typical reaction to these feelings is avoidance. When challenged by using your strength, fear gets smaller. Fearful men tend to focus on a bad, unsuccessful future. The antidote to this is to bring your full attention to the present by paying complete attention to your physical sensations, your feelings and sensations that are related to what is happening now. Give the present ALL of your attention and stay there as much as you can. This is not an exercise of perfection; we all must consider the future when we make plans and make choices. The future is a place we visit, whereas the present is where we live.

AVOIDANCE

Fear and anxiety are common expressed through the behavior of avoidance. When someone anticipates discomfort, the avoidance of that negative experience seems understandable and very human. However, the act of avoidance shows respect to fear which causes the fear to grow stronger and stronger. Avoidance interferes with life success and prevents achievement. If avoidance as a behavior pattern in a man's life occurs instead of taking responsibility, it will contribute to loss of his female partner's respect and admiration for him.

Avoidance appears in lack of responsibility-taking and patterns of procrastination. In both irresponsibility and procrastination, a man is not using his strength to challenge fear and adversity. In the cycle of performance anxiety where fear is high, a man may be acting out of patterns of sexual avoidance. Intercourse was temporarily suspended from your sex life to reduce fear and pressure, the potential for failure and to de-escalate patterns of avoidance.

ANGER

Become very aware of your anger-based feelings. Most people are unaware that anger-based feelings exist as a spectrum from low to high intensity. The only difference between them is the intensity. The low-intensity anger-based feelings are: annoyance, irritation, agitation, and frustration. Medium intensity anger-based feelings are: mad, upset, angry, heated, and pissed. High-intensity angry feelings are: enraged, rage, out-of-control, mayhem, and violent. Though different in intensity, all these feelings are anger-based.

We have angry feelings when an experience hurts us, blocks us, or interferes with the achievement of our goals and intentions. An angry feeling is energy mobilized to protect ourselves from a person or situation where we feel threatened. Anger is common and is in many ways a healthy emotion. It is not unusual that most days we have an experience that provokes our angry feelings. However, anger is part of an incomplete process. In anger, we are resisting an experience. By being angry, we are emotionally expressing, "No! I don't want this experience. I reject this." In anger, we oppose what is happening. Understandable! Many of our life experiences are not what we want. In most instances, our angry feelings are legitimate.

But angry feelings don't provide us with any benefits such as growth, improvements or progress. Being angry is a closed emotional state in which we are saying "No." Our life has other ideas. Our life, whether we like it or not, is saying we need these experiences, that is why the experience is in our life. A student may not like that he or she has a test, but his or her feelings about it don't matter. It only matters how the student responds and performs on the test. Angry feelings are like hating the test and refusing to take it while being the one who fails as a result!

Angry feelings only benefit us if we accept them, remain open and channel the energy mobilized by the anger to fix the problem, resolve the situation, grow from the experience. An alternative is to choose to be at peace by accepting the hardship. If we reject the experience by burying our angry feelings we lose at the game of life by not playing fully. We become blocked in our energy; we don't flow with life. Your problem with erections is a sign that you are refusing to participate

> If we reject an experience by burying our angry feelings without constructively using its energy, we lose at the game of life by not playing fully.

fully in life. Moving forward, adjust your attitude by accepting your angry feelings when you dislike something. Be open to it and inwardly say, "Yes, I am angry because I don't like what is happening. And I accept this as a challenge, and I am going to grow and learn from this by fixing the problem." When angry, there is a problem to be resolved.

If you only experience a small amount of anger, such as the low-intensity angry feelings, they are not less important than high-intensity anger, though they represent a less urgent problem. If you make attending to low-intensity angry feelings a priority by responding to them with solutions, you will be rewarded by a life that starts to be more and more positive and peaceful. If addressed quickly, small problems never grow into big ones. The more positive your life is, the less anger and anxiety you will have; important initial steps towards creating the positive environment that supports good erections and a satisfying sex life.

Practice identifying your feelings by apply words to each emotion you feel and express them, especially with your romantic partner so she understands you better. As you are able to positively and effectively interact with your feelings, you will start to feel confidence building. This is the development of emotional intelligence. The benefits to you go far beyond overcoming the breakdowns of performance anxiety. You will be better able to get support, be understood more, improve participation as a team member, improve the ability to solve problems, and will see improvements in your relationships, a foundation for better and more fulfilling sex.

STAYING IN THE PRESENT

The more you live in the present, the more satisfying and successful your life and sex life will be. The future is a place of fear, the past is

> The future is a place of fear. The past is a place of pain.
> The present is a place of freedom.

a place of pain, and the present is a place of freedom. A symptom of anxiety and living in the future is a busy mind. A busy mind can be uncomfortable and may have strong momentum that resists slowing. A helpful practice is to bring your attention to your body. Focus on your physical sensations while also checking your breathing to calm yourself. Exercise and meditation are healthy activities that help slow a busy mind. They also reduce the anxiety that causes it. We do not always have the power to stop the constant goals and deadlines of our future-oriented world, but we do have the power to stop our reactions so they don't take us over. As you pay attention to your emotions, you will notice that your feelings have a physical component. Increase your awareness of the full experience of your emotions and your body. Live in the present.

Emotional exercise 14: Have you felt any of the emotions listed above. Have you felt many feelings other than the ones mentioned? Do you handle angry feelings well? Do you tend to hold anger in? Have you ever exploded in anger? Take note of your patterns of avoidance. Are you good at expressing your feelings with words? Do you focus more on the future, the past or do you live mostly in the present? Write the answers to the questions in your journal. Continue to listen to the relaxation exercise daily.

Importance of Relationship Connection

The quality of your relationship influences your sexual performance greatly. In a moment of sexual play, how you feel about your sexual partner and how she feels about you impacts the quality of the moment and the quality of your play. As said previously, sex is holistic. Everything in your life gets included in sex because good sex requires complete openness. If you are only partially open, your sex has the potential to be partially good. If either you or your partner are harboring resentments, an intense sexual experience may awaken them. Most couples have experienced mechanical sex, all body, and with no emotional connection. The sex may feel good and may be satisfying physically, but it isn't fully dynamic and alive. When partners are angry or untrusting, they keep parts of themselves on the sidelines, unavailable for connection. The best sex includes fully open, all-in partners.

The connection between you and your partner is a large and influential factor. A positive connection that is open allows for great excitement which in turn helps your success at maintaining an erection. In the goal of setting yourself up for being a sexually functional and an effective lover, being aware of the quality of your love connection is valuable when evaluating whether or not intercourse is an activity at which you can be successful.

Look back upon your relationship and its history. Has your relationship been one that is mostly positive, peaceful, close and loving? Or has it been turbulent with many instances of anger, conflicts and hurtful moments? The emotional history of your relationship is encoded in the cells of you and your partner's bodies. The hurts and pain, if common, will be present in your lovemaking if not resolved. Some high-conflict couples attempt to make sex so active and intense to override their old pain, the same way a really loud noise may drown out a softer noise. This strategy can work in the moment but doesn't eliminate the reality of the problems. In the long run, it will not overcome the negative influence of pain within the relationship. The emotional quality of your relationship forms a foundation of how you and your partner feel about each other and affects your sexual play. A lot of hurt creates a shaky foundation that can easily undermine solid erections and the certainty of good sexual performance.

Events that are more recent have more influence over our prevailing emotional experience than those in the distant past. So if you and your lover are disconnected because of a series of minor conflicts during this past week, the after effects of the conflicts may interfere with a really good sexual connection. If you are stressed from overwhelming or upsetting workplace events, you may not be able to push through the anxiety that lingers. Is a problem troubling you which you cannot get out of your mind? These are small examples of situations when you cannot expect the best sexual performance from yourself. Your erection may be unreliable because of your uncomfortable emotions. Moving forward with intercourse under poor circumstances risks a poor outcome that may undo a lot of progress you have made towards your goal of escaping the cycle of performance anxiety.

> Moving forward with intercourse under poor circumstances risks a poor outcome.

Setting yourself up for success is sometimes accomplished by giving up on what you want most and accepting a choice with lower expectations and an assured positive outcome. Suggesting to your partner that you enjoy each other in non-intercourse ways of giving and receiving pleasure can avoid disappointment and setbacks. Of course, if sex progresses nicely, you feel relaxed within, you feel confident and have a solid stable erection, you may always suggest that intercourse is possible. (But only if the course has instructed you to re-integrate intercourse in your sex life.) Far better to under-promise and over-deliver than over-promise and disappoint. Protecting the moment from a negative experience avoids discomfort but more importantly, you will be protecting your partner from feeling bad. Helping your partner feel good is a high priority within your relationship and shows her she is important and valuable. Additionally, you will have given yourself a positive experience and avoided putting yourself in a negative position.

A healthy love relationship requires effort and regular investment of yourself, your time and your energy. If you don't put in enough effort, you will not get good results. A great comparison is a plant. It requires a certain amount of sunlight, fresh air, water, and good soil to survive. If those elements are present in sufficient quantities, the plant will grow. If one of the elements is missing, the plant may survive, but it will not thrive. If too many are missing the plant will inevitably die. If the necessary ingredients are missing, there is no amount of negotiating, begging or pleading with the plant to change the outcome. The plant will die. Love relationships are the same. If the necessary

> Relationships are incredibly honest, only the ones that are receiving the right amount of love, effort and time together will thrive.

ingredients are not present, the relationship or loving connection will die. Relationships are incredibly honest; only the ones that are receiving the right amount of love, effort and time together will thrive. If your relationship is troubled, the right amount of the vital ingredients are not present. No doubt about it.

The potential for a great sex life with healthy sexual functioning is maximized if your relationship is good, strong and satisfying. Sex may help to build a connection, but it is best to strengthen a connection that has already been built and is already strong. Sex is a great way to super-charge the connection. Using sexual and non-sexual methods to nourish your connection creates a strong balance. Eliminating negatives from the relationship may show the most dramatic improvements. Your romantic connection may be nourished by sharing yourself and your feelings with your partner, by working on a task or project together, and by spending relaxing quality time together. Being together in a new and unfamiliar environment may awaken those qualities in each of you that sparked your original attraction.

Affection is a distinct and vital form of relating. Loving through affectionate touch helps to energize and warm up the connection. A male tendency is to use loving touch as a way of initiating sex. However, affectionate touch is such an important form of loving that it must stand alone as a loving expression. Affectionate touch ought to be given generously, independent of any sexual intent. Moments are valuable when affection is shared which does not lead to sex. If never accomplished, a female partner may worry that sex is more important to her male partner than she is.

Keep your connection warm by spending time together which includes generous sharing, sensitivity to each other's feelings, and affectionate loving touch. By keeping the connection warm, you have a good launching pad from which to jump to "hot," the passionate intensity of lovemaking. A lack of negatives between you protects a close connection. A hurtful incident disproportionately harms the connection more than any loving gesture builds it. One hurt neutralizes the benefit of a dozen loving gestures. Not fair, but true. Generally, romantic partners are not sufficiently sensitive to each other's well-being to maintain a warm, positive connection, a truth that is worthy of consideration when making change.

TEAMMATES, FRIENDS AND LOVERS

Your efforts to generate a satisfying connection with your partner will happen differently in the three main phases of your relationship: teammates, friends, and lovers. As teammates, you and your partner communicate, coordinate, and synchronize so tasks are easily completed without frustration or negativity. By being good teammates, you can depend upon each other to do your part. Great teammates show consideration for the other's responsibilities by anticipating what the other must do. Each partner makes it easier by making efforts to reduce the other's work. Also as teammates, each of you can take initiative and accept responsibility by assuming the role of leader. When responsibility-taking is unbalanced, resentment may accumulate. Some men with a lot of anxiety are prone to avoidance, procrastination and not taking responsibility. Stepping up by assuming a strong, adult role in your relationship is part of building pride in yourself and a happy partner. Other anxious men seek to have a lot of control as a way to reduce uncertainty. Balancing shared control may help to reduce negativity for the partner.

As friends, partners share themselves. Friendship is the core of a love relationship. It is characterized by a positive emotional connection. Best friends know everything about each other, which reinforces strong trust. Partners are open to each other. They show compassion and sensitivity which supports understanding. As friends, partners the sharing of deeply held feelings builds a positive emotional connection. A good friendship includes a close connection. Closeness is an essential ingredient in a solid friendship. The emotional awareness exercises will strengthen your ability to participate in a closer friendship connection. Good friends enjoy spending time together and laugh a lot when relaxed; they are sensitive to each other's well-being. They support each other and make each other's life better because they are together. Male partners prize the vital component of loyalty; partners having each other's back. Female partners prioritize both sharing and support.

When partners act insensitively and do not understand each other, the friendship is diminished. If the status of the friendship between romantic partners has eroded or died, it may cause the sexual relationship to disappear. Female partners tend to experience sex as unsupported without a good friendship connection. If absent of friendship, the connection between you and your partner will not support arousal and maintained erections.

Finally, romantic partners are lovers. You are very aware of the importance of sex in your relationship. You are also acutely aware of how harmful a troubled sex life can be. At its best, when a couple is strong sexually, partners feel joy at giving each other sexual pleasure. Partners act as a team to build excitement. They may explore each other's eroticism in varied fantasy play. If sex is imbalanced between partners' desires, interests, type of sexual play, etc., sex can become a negative force in the relationship.

When performance anxiety has caused damage, some male partners turn to masturbation and porn (erotic or fantasy material) for sexual satisfaction, sexual activity with little risk of erection failure. But many female partners are threatened and hurt by the use of porn. Most women feel that porn use is a form of cheating. Covert porn use, if discovered, adds a layer of deception on top of the pain of betrayal. This can further pollute a couple's sex life and harm their status as lovers. Through this course, you should develop an understanding between you about what form masturbation may take to avoid hurtfulness. Openness and communication about it help.

Emotional exercise 15: Write in your journal about the quality of your relationship connection. Does it add positively to your life or negatively affect your life? In what ways does your relationship connection help or harm your level of confidence? Discuss the amount of affectionate touch between you. Does your relationship connection support a good sexual relationship and your arousal? How strong is your relationship in the phases of teammates, friends and lovers? Discuss your observations with your partner.

Sexual exercise 10: How reliable have your erections been during partner sex? Have you felt any anxiety? If so, have you been able to calm it? If your 30 second intervals of intercourse have gone well, and you are relaxed as well as comfortable, expand intercourse to a minute, if the quality of the moment supports it. During any moments of distraction or negative feeling, if your erection softens, don't panic. Discontinue intercourse while redirecting your focus to pleasuring your partner or receiving pleasure in a different way until you feel more positive and more relaxed. If successful, you may attempt intercourse again if your erection returns and your partner is receptive.

The Rigors of Relating

Loving another person is among the hardest life goals to undertake. People hope to be lucky in love, but luck has little to do with

> The quality of your love for yourself directly determines how effective you will be at loving another.

romantic success. We are attracted to and choose a partner not based on luck but based on our emotional history and our inner relationship with ourselves. The well-worn statement about loving yourself first is spot on. The quality of your love for yourself directly determines how effective you will be at loving another. Our personalities are made of many layers, most of which are unconscious.

The deeper layers are older and have been covered over as you have grown and aged. The layers contain unhealed wounds, sources of pain, and great unhappiness; they will affect your capacity to be open and to love.

When we connect with another person, as the relationship ages and deepens, and the importance of the romantic partner increases, the love penetrates many of your inner emotional layers. It awakens the painful emotions stored there. The old feelings that have been activated influence your personality. In a new relationship, this is the process of the fading of the honeymoon period. In established relationships, it is the difficulties that infect loving partners which complicate the loving connection. It is a normal process of healing, but it makes life and love very difficult. These old feelings are painful. The process of healing is painful. While healing is positive, it doesn't feel positive. Loving another pins us against our very own weaknesses and wounds. The very fibers of our being are tested. This is what makes loving another the most difficult challenge we may ever undertake.

Romantic partners experience disappointment as the process of what may have been tremendous love becomes the painful reality that, "You are not who I thought you were." Love relationships are, in reality, the work of growing and healing. For many partners, the rigors of a relationship may cause it to feel like it is "more than I bargained for." As the deeper issues are brought to the surface, partners are also likely to express that, "This is not what I signed up for." But in actuality, the process is exactly what both partners signed up for because it is an expression of each partner's unique path of growth.

As old pain arises in the psyches of both partners, tension, conflict, adversity, and disconnection replace the close, loving connection. It is painful. It is disappointing. For men who develop erectile dysfunction and get trapped by the cycle of performance anxiety, the old feelings that have been awakened show up as anxiety, fear, powerlessness, and avoidance. These are the difficult emotions that form the problem of performance anxiety.

The manner in which the partners relate and how they handle their pain makes the difference between a compassionate connection where partners are mutually supportive or an adversarial connection that is combative. When both partners feel deep pain, they are at risk for selfish choices and behaviors. People in pain have difficulty being open and attentive to others. If you and your partner cope poorly with the pain, it will exacerbate the problem of performance anxiety. Successful couples are skilled problem-solving teams. Successful couples, when they have a problem they make it smaller, unsuccessful couples make problems bigger.

In your relationship, if pain results in critical, hurtful, attacking, accusatory, contemptuous, or disrespectful behaviors and attitudes, then the dynamics are giving life and energy to performance anxiety. Without reducing and eliminating these negative tendencies, the patterns of performance anxiety will not be reduced. Failed erections are an expression of both individual and relationship pain.

Make every effort to break the connection between your pain and negative treatment of your partner. Use all your strength to show love, in all its forms. Your motivations for a loving attitude need not be determined by your feelings for your partner, which may be mixed or negative during difficult times. Instead, choose to behave out of your love and respect for yourself. Behave in a way that is your best, so that at minimum, you may be proud of yourself. By doing so, you are being part of your relationship's solution instead of perpetuating the problems. Unresolved problems perpetuate pain and may interfere with the resolution of your symptoms of performance anxiety.

For the Partner

We have already discussed how the onset of erectile dysfunction of performance anxiety is interpreted by female partners as a lack of attraction. For her, the pain of this realization may be substantial. It may be carried by her for months and even years. We briefly touched on different ways that female partners react during sex when her man's erection withers.

The way she responds to her male partner and how she relates to him has a large influence. A relationship is a system. Partners influence each other. So a man's chance of improving his sexual functioning is unlikely if he does not feel supported by his female partner. To reiterate: he may be the one with the problem, but his female partner must be part of the solution. Without her assistance, his efforts at escaping the cycle of performance anxiety are doomed. Truly, it is the couple that must be repaired, not just the man. Even in a relationship where she does not feel important, a female partner is highly influential. She is important and her contributions are essential. To improve his love, the male partner must show her that she is important in many small and large ways.

> He may be the one with the problem, but his female partner must be part of the solution.

When a male partner is unable to maintain his erection, he is highly aware of the impact on his female partner. The way she responds will not be able to fix or prevent the problem, but her actions may complicate and even prevent the solution. Critical, accusatory, attacking, shaming, or blaming expressions hurt a male partner in an already uncomfortable and vulnerable state. Hurtful reactions are not just a momentary lack of compassion, they add pain on top of pain and will make repairing the situation exponentially more difficult. Such behavior is far less than her best and will prevent pride in herself in addition to a poor quality relationship and sex life.

As a rule, in a healthy love relationship, partners are sensitive and compassionate to each other's pain. But when a partner is also in pain, compassion is more difficult to give to the other. When both partners are simultaneously in pain, a lot of emotional strength is required to avoid escalated conflict. In the situation of a failed erection, a female partner is well served by putting her own hurt, frustration, and disappointment to the side and offering compassionate attention to her male partner. She maintains a delicate balance; quiet compassion is a kind offering. However, if it sounds to her man like she pities him or is patronizing, he may be further hurt and react in anger.

Upon losing his erection, if he has not withdrawn or shut down, she may still engage with him. By gentling acknowledging his failure with a hopeful message of togetherness, such as "We will get through this," she shows support and teammate-like loyalty. Holding him tightly in a compassionate embrace may help. If she signals that she is ready to engage in non-intercourse pleasuring, it is a message that she chooses not to dwell on the failure and instead is ready to move on in loving him.

Recognize that due to the painful failure from which he is hurting, nothing may work if the male partner gives in to his pain by becoming emotionally shut down. At an awkward and delicate moment, the goal is to avoid making the situation worse and to maximize the possibility that repair of the sexual session may occur. By showing support, the female partner also helps lower the risk that the moment's pain provokes anger or conflict. There will be scenarios where there just is no winning. Once the two of you have begun working to escape from the cycle of performance anxiety, the way you respond should become less awkward and more assured as you two progress. Hopefully, it will soon start to feel less like a crisis and more like a situation you know how to handle.

FOR THE PARTNER IN RELATING

A female partner is important and ought to be treated as such. As already said, she is highly influential. Whether she uses her power or not, she is powerful. Her happiness, satisfaction, admiration, and loyalty are deeply valued and desired by her male partner. Unless a relationship is toxic, polluted with damaged trust, bitterness and resentment, she has some power to be a part of the solution. With her influence and love, a female partner may help create an environment that supports the best relationship. Along the way, she may use the adversity to better herself, while creating a better relationship and a better sex life while escaping from the cycle of performance anxiety as a couple.

How she participates as a teammate in problem-solving may make issues smaller or larger. How she relates to her male partner may foster his growth or erode his confidence. Love relationships and marriages are incredibly difficult; they test us thoroughly. In times of adversity, do you control your difficult emotions well, or do you release them intensely upon your male partner in moments of frustration? Are you supportive and kind or critical and berating? Expressing intense emotions with a sharp, raised voice with an angry attitude is experienced as disrespectful by male partners. It will contribute to the erosion of his confidence. As an alternative, letting him know softly and gently that you need something different from him is superior. Men tend to react to high emotional intensity with withdrawal, avoidance, defensiveness and counter-attacking. He must learn to

> Expressing intense emotions at him in a sharp loud way with angry attitude will be felt by him as disrespectful and will contribute to the erosion of his confidence.

react in improved ways, but you may help by expressing yourself more effectively at producing a better result.

How do you cope with your anxious feelings? If your anxiety is expressed with controlling words and actions that rob your male partner of choice in the relationship, then you may be unintentionally and indirectly contributing to an environment that results in performance anxiety. A female partner is never the cause of her male partner's inability to maintain his erection, but she can contribute to his success in sex and life or undermine it. Well-defined boundaries between partners are consistent with each partner feeling free to be accepted for who he or she is. Well-respected boundaries also help to maintain an equal and balanced distribution of power between you and your partner. If how you relate adds to power imbalance, disrespect, and build-up of resentment, your efforts to alter these patterns for the better will be necessary. Eliminating performance anxiety from the relationship is helped by a reduction of tension, conflict, negativity and all other relationship issues. Your efforts are needed towards this goal.

As his romantic partner, you deserve the best: great love, to be cherished, to be honored, and to be celebrated. But you will not have these if you are not proud enough of yourself to believe you deserve them. If your partner does not treat you well, you must demand better. Strive to be the person you can be proud of. Be careful to avoid hurtfulness to yourself, your partner, and others. Hurtful behavior will undermine being loved in the best way. Such behavior indirectly makes solving the sexually-based difficulties in the relationship harder.

When partners are unable to eliminate or reduce factors that cause tension, conflict, and negativity in the relationship, couples therapy may be a necessary step to make vital growing changes and adjustments. Positive conditions are necessary to resolve the symptoms of performance anxiety.

Emotional exercise 16: Initiate a discussion with your partner. Listen to her with a goal of understanding (not necessarily also agreeing) without interrupting to learn if she feels important to you. Ask her what adjustments she is willing to make to contribute to the resolution of performance anxiety. Learn from her about her needs, both filled and unfulfilled, in the relationship. Be ready to use your strength to make growing improvements.

A Man's Relationship with Himself

Self-esteem is the bedrock upon which a man's successes and failures rest. In the case of erectile dysfunction within the cycle of performance anxiety, the man's level of self-esteem is central. On the outside, his confidence may look solid, but open the hood and you will see an engine that is not firing on all cylinders. Every man and woman alike can benefit from growth. The development of performance anxiety has revealed the weak areas where your growth is most needed.

> The development of performance anxiety has revealed the area in which your growth is most needed.

Most men who succumb to performance anxiety have lived with anxiety-related difficulties most of their lives. Many of them grew up in families where one or both parents also suffered from anxiety and related issues. Life with anxiety isn't easy and men who routinely feel fear are at odds with the values of the masculine ideal. In the masculine ideal, there is no allowance for weaknesses, fear, and anxiety. Buried deep in his psyche is a sense of failure and shame that he could never be a real man because he feels much fear and anxiety.

His reaction to his perceived shortcomings is likely have lasted for decades in the forms of self-rejection, self-disrespect, and regular self-disappointment. These aspects of the negative relationship he has with himself and the shame that comes along with them are evident in the current symptoms of performance anxiety. Yet, the struggle for self-esteem and pride have no bearing on the man's real capacity and worth. He has rejected himself before his real worth could be proven.

The devastation from being unable to fulfill a man's primal duty of satisfying a female partner may prove to be his final indignity before taking a courageous step to overcome his anxiety and low self-esteem. If you get the right help, which I hope will be this course, getting trapped in the cycle of performance anxiety may result in finally breaking through your self-rejection to learning that you are truly good and worthy. Your worth will not be proven by your restored ability to maintain your erection, but from healing the long-standing negative self-esteem underneath and finally growing beyond it.

LOVING YOURSELF

Having an improved relationship with yourself will be a requirement for your success. It starts with your internal dialogue, the inner conversation that constitutes your thoughts. In that dialogue, there is the part of you that speaks and the part of you that listens. This is the conversation between "me" and "myself." When self-esteem is low, the inner dialogue has a negative quality, possibly even harsh, insulting, demeaning and hurtful. Disrespectful language may be used when you are angry with yourself. The inner attitude can be one of rejection and failure such as calling yourself a loser. Having a negative self-relationship will undermine your success in growing and improving.

When a poor self-relationship is present, a man has unrealistic expectations for himself that he fails to achieve. As the cycle of failures and inner self-abuse rages, a negative cycle similar to the cycle of performance anxiety is energized. The more hateful you are to yourself, the more you disappoint yourself, the further your self-hate is fueled. It is a downward spiral. Your dark view of yourself may be about your anxiety and the many situations in which it has overpowered your success at achieving goals and ambitions. Instead of achievements, a cycle of self-disappointment is created.

Improving the relationship with yourself will be accomplished by cleaning up your inner world. In your inner dialogue, you will benefit from making the relationship between the thinking and the listening, between "me" and "myself," a gentler, kinder more positive relationship. Inwardly, lowering your intensity and gradually reducing your anxiety by cultivating more patience and self-acceptance is the right effort. The way you think about and to yourself is better if it is supportive and gentle, like the attitude you expect from a good friend or your romantic partner. Striking a balance inwardly between being kind and patient with yourself while also holding yourself accountable. Demand of yourself your best efforts, but do so without negativity, disrespect, or harshness. Mistakes are normal. Your mistakes are beneficial when they are part of our learning, but we cannot learn if we are attacked for mistakes. If mistakes happen under threat of punishment, they are viewed only as failures. We are not perfect, we are human. Mistakes must be accepted as part of your learning process. Henry Link said, "While one person hesitates because he feels inferior, the other is busy making mistakes and becoming superior."

A healthy and positive inner dialogue is achievable through practice. It takes time. Watching for the quality expressed in the attitude of your thoughts, such as negative, angry, disrespectful, demanding, berating or insulting. These are the kinds of thoughts that are ripe for improvement. Imagine if your thoughts were how a three-year-old child was talking to you. Undoubtedly you wouldn't tolerate a child talking to you in a demanding or insulting manner. Gently but firmly say to yourself, "Say that again, but say it more nicely this time." Clean up your thoughts by insisting that they are positive and suitable for being said out loud in a place of worship, in front of your mother, or your children. By treating yourself kindly, you are being a better friend to yourself.

INTEGRITY

In an effort to improve your relationship with yourself, practice operating with high integrity. You may be thinking, "What does integrity have to do with my erection?" The focus of this section is upon the depths of a solid foundation being built to develop resiliency, the ability to tolerate emotional challenges without erection failure. You benefit from possessing strength in a variety of forms: emotional resiliency,

> Integrity is the practice of holding tightly to good values, such as being non-hurtful, honest and dependable without surrendering them, even during challenging times.

stability, emotional regulation and impulse control, to succeed under many difficult circumstances. Acting with integrity requires effort which benefits you by reducing your anxiety and while developing a feeling of pride. Integrity is the practice of maintaining good values, such as being non-hurtful, honest, reliable and dependable even during challenging times. By being consistently careful with your word, by being true to your word, your life and relationship becomes simpler and of better quality. When you demonstrate integrity, you will be earning your partner's trust and respect, as well as your own self-respect. Mutual respect is a great feeling that supports your ability to relax when an opportunity to be intimate arrives.

RESPONSIBILITY AND OWNERSHIP

No one is more responsible for the quality of your life than you. The concepts of ownership and taking responsibility refer to a kind of masculine maturity where you own your power and not reduce it by not seeking to blame others. Shirking responsibility is a bad habit that prevents the development of masculine power. By accepting responsibility, you allow your life and all that is in it, good and bad, success or failure, to be an expression of yourself. Ownership signifies that if something is in your life, you receive it as challenge you will accept, to take care of so that your life, your partner's and your family's life is good. Taking ownership is the opposite of ignoring and avoiding. Once you own your life and circumstances fully, deceiving yourself is gone and in its place is the power to grow, learn, and improve. Your mistakes are a valuable part of you, but you cannot benefit from them if you avoid responsibility.

Another unhealthy value of the masculine myth is the belief that failure is not an option. If we are strong enough to take a risk, sometimes we will fail. If we possess healthy confidence, instead of blaming others or circumstances, we own our failures and mistakes by learning from them so they are not repeated. Ownership and taking responsibility are essential ingredients in the development of leadership. Little expresses confidence and masculine power more than leadership. Strength, power, and leadership are male qualities that are highly attractive to and a turn-on for female partners. As you own your power, you will also own the power to make your life better, including your sex life.

THE QUEEN AND THE KING

The distinction between an authentic, strong and confident man and a "real man" is knowing how to love. The authentic man has substance. The "real man" is a concept and an ideal that lives more in movies and in imaginations than in daily life. Loving yourself, your partner, others, and life effectively makes you a strong and confident man. Your love relationship is the place to practice loving. Your female partner is not a perfect being, but like yourself, she is a human being.

> Loving yourself, your partner, others and life effectively makes you strong and confident.

Loving her is essential even in moments when her limitations are on display. Doing so means possessing the strengths of acceptance, forgiveness, and patience. The degree to which you treat your female partner like a queen is a measure of your masculine power, how able you are to love, honor and cherish her. A strong and confident man treats his woman well at all times. Simultaneously, your woman ought to treat you like a king, with respect and admiration. As you grow by loving yourself more and more, you make it increasingly easier for your female partner to give you the royal treatment.

Emotional exercise 17: What did you notice about the feelings you felt as you read this section? To what degree have you possessed the strengths discussed in this section? What are the strengths and practices that will help you to live better while liking yourself and your life more? Have you noticed parts of your life where you can take more responsibility and ownership? List these in your journal.

Letting Go

As men, we easily identify with the qualities of strength and power. Men have a seemingly natural tendency to respond to all situations with force. This is manifested in many small and large ways such as conflict, fixing something that is broken, or punishing a child for bad behavior. As men, our inflexibility has been mentioned in several

> As men, our tendency to be inflexible and single-minded contributed to the development of performance anxiety.

instances before, our pattern to address situations in a single-minded way by using power, by taking action without considering other possibilities. Our female partners can see more clearly options other than the ones we choose; they grow frustrated that we choose methods that may not be the best fit for a situation. As men, our tendency to be inflexible and single-minded contributes to the development of performance anxiety.

Earlier in the course, we explored the skill of relaxing. You have been listening to the relaxation exercise for days or weeks by this point. If you have succeeded in relaxing yourself, you have learned that part of that skill is that of letting go. To relax, you have been releasing all that occupies you and all that you hold on to. Letting go is a necessary and vital skill; it is the opposite of using force. You use this skill on a daily basis when you go to sleep, another instance of letting go. Overcoming performance anxiety will require you to make letting go a strength. Letting go of fear and anxiety are obvious examples.

A secure man can step to the side in the right moments. Emotional security is similar to and part of confidence. A variation of letting go is getting out of the way. Insecure men are those who have not developed confidence; they inwardly fear that they are not valuable. When a man has a low sense of worth, he will see others, including his romantic partner, highlighting his worthlessness in their actions and choices whether or not they are truly doing so. As a result, these men have trouble getting out of their own way. They insert themselves into situations in which their presence and participation are unnecessary and not helpful. They have a blindness in which not participating touches their pain of worthlessness. The outcome is over-complications which leads to troubles that could have been avoided.

Men with low worth look for opportunities to prove their value, but their motivation is about themselves instead of the larger goal. Oftentimes, less is more. Many situations will resolve with little or no action or involvement, an observation visible only to a secure man. Letting go by getting out of our own way helps to keep the quality of life high. Patience is a strength in which letting go is active. Listening also is a skill in which letting go is required. Understanding is accomplished by letting go. Sometimes a good outcome is produced is by choosing to wait instead of habitually doing more. Men who respond in a single-minded way to most situations by using force miss opportunities to be a good friend to themselves.

PRESSURE AND FORCE

Using pressure and force is an expression that reveals a closed emotional state. We assert our will in using pressure and force. Being sensitive and receptive are open states. When we are open, we have the potential to respond in tune to the needs of the moment. Getting caught in the trap of performance anxiety and the resulting erection loss was an attempt to use pressure and force when their use was ineffective and insensitive to the moment. You probably use this ineffective strategy in other places in your life as well. By being conscious of your tendencies, you may improve by considering openness instead of being closed. When force and pressure are used where a more open strategy is appropriate, damage is done. Within your relationship with your female partner, loving efforts are best, the use of force and pressure will damage emotional trust and safety. To love well, openness is required. We cannot succeed at loving if we are closed. Being open is possible only by routinely letting go.

"ONE-WAY" THINKING

For most men, an inflexible and "one-way" mindset is unconscious. Ask them about it and they will deny its existence. A blind spot is complete when we do not know what we do not know. Men are not routinely aware of their failures because they blame others or the situation for the breakdown. Female partners can see their man's single-mindedness clearly, and they suffer for it as well. An inflexible man will not want to hear his female partner's perspective out of concern that doing so may make him look wrong or stupid. In actuality, considering additional perspectives is commonly quite a smart move which increases the odds of a good outcome.

Men react to situations in terms of how they must act or what they must do. Many men are ready to inflexibly oppose anything as if it is the arrival of an enemy. However, opposition is a closed state with limited options. Opposing a situation invites conflict and drama. In conflict, both sides lose while attempting to gain a victory. Opposing a partner will create drama and hurt. When partners argue, the relationship and both partners always lose. The practice of acceptance is a peaceful, open reaction that offers a large chance of a good outcome. Again, less is more. Acceptance is practiced by letting go of fear, anger and the desire to control circumstances.

CONTROL

Control is fear's agent. In moments when you feel afraid or anxious, controlling the environment may seem like a natural way to feel better. If it has been a life-long pattern of behavior you may not be conscious that you are using control. As a method of moderating your own inner experience, control becomes one of the inflexible and single-minded methods of using power and force that does not serve you. In your love relationship, if your partner feels controlled, she will identify this as a negative element that interferes with her feeling loved by you. It is better to calm and soothe your fear within yourself than to need to control others or your environment.

> In your love relationship, if your partner feels controlled she will identify this as a negative that interferes with her feeling loved by you.

Letting go is a natural strength. When you breathe, your inhale is healthy only if it is followed by an exhale. Exhaling is letting go. You will only be able to move forward to new opportunities by letting go of old ones. You will only be successful at overcoming performance anxiety by letting go of the pain and memories of your past sexual disappointments. Letting go of fear and anger will be of prime importance in your success. In addition to challenging fear, letting go of it is needed at times as well. Your anger represents a test of your ability to redirect your angry energy to a solution, but sometimes letting go of your anger can be useful in not allowing a bad event, one that has angered you, from creating unnecessary hardship. The practice of acceptance may transform anger into peace. That is a form of letting go. Another form of it is simply letting go of the anger while you choose to move on to the next life event. You maintain your power by letting go in this way. Loosening the grip of performance anxiety is through your ability to let go.

Emotional exercise 18: Do you identify any of these tendencies in your thinking or behavior? Start to practice letting go of these tendencies. In your journal, write down moments when you succeeded at letting go of control, pressure, and one-way thinking. When you have successfully let go, what was the result?

Sexual exercise 11: Re-evaluate your sexual experiences. Are you feeling more confident about your erections? Have you had any successes? If you are feeling positive, less anxious, and more confident, are you ready to extend intercourse to two minutes? Make this choice based on knowing yourself and your feelings. Make the choice to expand intercourse based upon the wisdom of setting yourself up for success. It is a success if you are not ready and you decide to delay extending the duration of intercourse. Know your limits. Not every sexual session needs to include intercourse. However, it is best that every experience of sex includes love, connection, closeness, fun, and pleasure.

Contributing Factors

We are complex beings. Our lives are complicated with dozens of responsibilities, details and requirements. The more that we love; ourselves, our partners, others and life, the more our lives gradually become simplified. Until then, consider the many factors which may negatively impact you and contribute to getting trapped in the cycle of performance anxiety. Identifying them may help you in understanding yourself better and even become empowered to escape the trap. Until now, you may have noticed that the self-fulfilling prophecy has elements that are obvious contributors, but as this course has progressed, you have become increasingly familiar with the deep and large foundation of factors that are underneath.

Many of the contributing factors may apply to you and your relationship whereas others are more specialized and may be relevant to only a select few, but still warrant being addressed. As you read through, even if the issues do not apply to you, learning about them will further your understanding of human functioning.

SEXUAL FACTORS

Sex is a part of being human. It is as natural and normal as eating and breathing. While we will not die without sex as we would if we stopped breathing or eating, sex is obviously of great importance. Eating and breathing do not generate the same kind of buzz that sex does. Sex is controversial, edgy, dirty, and thrilling and therefore comes with a lot of ambivalence and baggage. Throughout history, sex has been regarded with a suspicion that has come from its associated with carnal desires and sinfulness. The carnal natured of sex has caused it to be associated with a widespread ambivalence and contrary nature in which good and bad flip flop, such as in the phrase, "You are a really *bad* boy!" can mean that you are an exciting or skilled lover. The same sense that sex is bad has pervaded our culture in the form of sexual shame. It is unfortunately common. For too many, bodies and sex parts are the source of embarrassment, discomfort and shame. Varying sex acts bump into sexual partners' discomfort. As we have already discussed, sex and our sexual selves operate best in a relaxed and positive environment. When painful feelings pollute the sexual arena, other uncomfortable feelings will be generated, such as frustration, anxiety, disappointment, disconnection and sexual dysfunction, including erection unreliability or loss.

PAST ABUSE

A tragic truth is that many men and women have experienced the trauma of physical abuse, sexual abuse, childhood sexual abuse and violence. These can permanently scar a person emotionally. The impact of past abuse on a couple can play a huge and complicating factor in the attempt to have a positive and satisfying sex life. Many partners who have been damaged by past abuse, and the couple in which they are a part, are unsuccessful at getting beyond the intense fear-based reactions that are triggered by sex.

Men who experienced past sexual abuse are likely to have many mixed feelings about sex and their sexual selves. Sex may feel like a overwhelming and uncomfortable minefield that is best avoided. Female partners who have been harmed by abuse are unfortunately more common than men and may also display patterns of avoidance and discomfort with sex. Some abused men may have no sexual desire, ambivalence in sexual preference, routines of sexual avoidance, and erectile dysfunction that looks a lot like performance anxiety. Even though the source of the erectile dysfunction is similar, including forms of fear and anxiety, in cases of past abuse and sexual abuse the process of healing the pain is more complex than simple anxiety-based performance anxiety. If trauma-based factors are regularly an obstacle to satisfying closeness and intimacy, working with a skilled therapist will be necessary.

EJACULATORY CONTROL PROBLEMS

Other sexual complications may be roadblocks in your quest to be a great sexual couple. At its best, sex is positive. Any negativity will dampen your potential for great excitement, high pleasure, and amazing connection. Many men are troubled by ejaculatory control problems in addition to performance anxiety. The two may be interwoven. Problems with ejaculation may cause performance anxiety or the reverse. One may cause a reoccurrence of the other or form an obstacle to repairing the other.

The most common ejaculatory control problem is premature ejaculation or ejaculating before a man wishes to or intends to. At its worst, men ejaculate even before entering their female partner. This dysfunction leads to shame, disappointment, frustration, and feelings of inadequacy. Other men can begin intercourse but ejaculate much sooner than they prefer or intend, after only a few seconds. Female partners share in the painful feelings, typically of disappointment and frustration. Premature ejaculation may form a self-fulfilling cycle that is equal to that of erectile dysfunction. Men who have difficulty with ejaculatory control also often have a challenge of anxiety and low self-esteem, both as a cause of and a result of the problem.

Men who ejaculate too soon will benefit from reduced anxiety and greater awareness of the physical sensations within their bodies. When a man is highly anxious, he has reduced physical awareness. Slowing down excitement is part of the solution practiced during masturbation, but then gradually introduced into couple play. Another ejaculatory control problem is delayed or absent ejaculation. Men with the inability to slow down the arrival of orgasm may wish they had the problem of delayed ejaculation. But while it may seem better, it is equally a problem. Some men are embarrassed and troubled by ejaculation that takes too long or even cannot be reached. In their embarrassment, they may make excuses or even fake orgasm to hide their limitation.

Delayed ejaculation occurs when a man has difficulty reaching orgasm. He is unsuccessful at ejaculating during intercourse or has to try hard to ejaculate, but eventually succeeds. Some couples place a premium on the overly high expectation of simultaneous orgasm during intercourse. The couples who succeed and regularly experience this are the exception. The unrealistic goal of simultaneous orgasm may set couples up for sexual-based problems because of the pressure partners may use to create success. A man with delayed ejaculation does not orgasm when his female partner does. Oftentimes men have to thrust vigorously to finish while their female partner remains inactive. Other couples will use manual stimulation or self-stimulation after intercourse.

Inhibited ejaculation happens when a man is unable to ejaculate at all. Both forms of ejaculatory control problems have a silver lining, though most men plagued by the problem do not appreciate it. Inhibited ejaculation can be caused by the pressure men put on themselves to succeed, often because they value their female partner's satisfaction over their own. Men who have trouble with taking too long have great lasting power which may benefit their female partner if she prefers long duration intercourse. The downside to it is that her man may require intercourse to last too long beyond her arousal. If a man persists in trying to reach orgasm beyond his female partner's arousal and her lubrication has disappeared, soreness and discomfort may result.

Similar to performance anxiety, female partners may react to delayed or inhibited ejaculation by taking his limitation personally, as evidence that she is not attractive enough, desirable, or loved. The collateral difficulties caused by this share similarities with the damage caused by the erection failure in performance anxiety. Men may get trapped in a cycle that contributes to patterns and repetitions of the problem. However, neither delayed nor inhibited ejaculation are problems unless the man or couple make them so. If a man is unable to reach orgasm but is fine with it and his female partner has no negative reaction, then it is not a problem.

Among the causes of both forms of ejaculation problems are a man's tendency to put too much pressure on himself. Doing so may be an expression of anxiety-based issues. In many cases, a man wants to please his female partner so much that he pressures himself to succeed resulting in the development of an ejaculation problem. Reducing and eliminating pressure is part of the solution. The cycle is also energized by a man's one-way attitude; that force is the only way to respond to a problem. He believes that if a little force doesn't succeed, more force will be better. In the dilemma of delayed or inhibited ejaculation, when a man puts pressure on himself his ejaculation will be difficult to obtain, but when he ramps up the pressure ejaculation may become impossible. In the case of diminishing returns, the more he tries, the less he succeeds.

DISCREPANCY OF SEXUAL DESIRE

When a wheel is unbalanced, the more that it is used without correction, the more unbalanced it becomes. This simple concept applies to every problem a couple has. Because couples are strengthened by equal and mutual loving, the exchange of love forms a cycle. When an imbalance occurs, such as performance anxiety or any other sustained stress or strain, without strength and resiliency, a couple will have difficulty adjusting, adapting, or correcting it. The discrepancy of

> The greater the difference between partners the more difficult is achieving a resolution.

sexual desire is an imbalance in the frequency which partners value and prefer sex. When one partner wishes for a greater frequency of sex than the other, because sex always includes our core values and the necessity of being true to ourselves, this imbalance may be resistant to successful negotiation. The greater the difference between partners the more difficulty in achieving a resolution. Unresolved, the pain from this issue may contaminate the entire relationship, similar to the way the toxic emotion from performance anxiety may have grown in your relationship. The negatives generated by the discrepancy of sexual desire have the potential to kick off other dysfunctions, such as erection problems with the cycle of performance anxiety.

A variation on a theme of discrepancy is that of sexual interest. Tension and disconnection may result from partners who have very different ideas about what constitutes satisfying sex. Partners naturally vary in many ways. Partners in a healthy relationship share many interests, but no two people want the same thing in the same amount, in the same way, at the same time all the time. We are unique and so are our sexual preferences. Our eroticism of how we express love is unique like our fingerprint. Because sex represents a wide spectrum of activities, many of which are desired due to underlying aspects of our eroticism, sometimes an activity that is interesting, exciting and a turn-on to one partner is a turn-off or crosses the line into unacceptability to the other. The discrepancy of sexual interests, if unresolved, may produce accumulated negative emotions, such as resentment, distrust and disconnection.

DESIRE

Partner differences extend to desire for sex as well as the desire for anything else. When the partners' level of desire varies widely, negative feelings are generated. The situation is particularly difficult when a partner feels little or no sexual desire. Instead of the problem being a discrepancy of desire, it is considered a disorder of desire. The negative feelings between partners provoked by a lack of desire can be substantial. Sexual desire is a complex human quality that arises from many factors such as self-esteem, the degree to which a person feels empowered, the quality of relationship connection, history of upbringing, and many factors including every physical system of the body. Resurrecting desire can therefore be complex. Determining the source of the cause may be like an investigation. Unresolved, the negative impact on a partner and love relationship has the power to provoke other relationship problems, such as tension and conflict and sexual problems, such as erection loss and getting stuck in the cycle of performance anxiety.

By this point, you may have noticed a pattern. Any unresolved problem, whether personal, relational, or sexual, may contribute to the creation of other problems. Whenever several systems are interdependent, problem transmission is possible. For instance, if a car is driving for a long time with unbalanced wheels, eventually the car's suspension may become damaged and eventually by a failure of the stabilizing structure and ultimately can cause the exhaust system to malfunction. Our emotional, relationship and sexual lives are interdependent and therefore vulnerable to problem transmission.

ORGASM

At the peak of pleasure is orgasm. No experience is more sought after. An orgasm isn't just about pleasure; the openness demonstrated by a climaxing partner reassures a lover of love. An orgasm also signals to a partner who is insecure in his or her sexual skills that he or she has loved skillfully. But not all partners reach orgasm. A high number of couples suffer from unrealistic expectations that arise from a lack of sexual information and education. As mentioned earlier in this section, some male partners suffer from inhibited orgasm. Female partners may also be challenged this way. Roughly one-third of women have not yet become orgasmic. Another third of women achieve orgasm, not during intercourse but through manual, oral, or vibrator stimulation. The final third achieves orgasm during intercourse some of the time. Most women do not achieve orgasm consistently through intercourse, though small percentage of exceptional women do. Theory suggests that if determined, every woman can learn to be orgasmic, and with practice most women can be orgasmic during intercourse. Additionally, most men and women can develop the skill of multiple orgasms. But for those who have yet to become orgasmic, the absence of climax can add strain and stress to a couple's sex life, especially when the partner's emotional security is dependent upon orgasmic success. Unresolved, the disorder can accumulate negativity which may contribute to the development of male performance anxiety and other sexual and relationship problems.

VAGINISMUS

A very difficult female problem is vaginismus. Sexual problems are pain magnets. The emotional distress caused by sexual difficulty easily spreads and painfully affects the whole relationship. Vaginismus is an emotionally-based disorder in which a woman is afraid of penetration of intercourse and as a result, tightens her pelvic muscles in anticipation of pain. The condition is demonstrated along a spectrum of severity. At its least, a woman experiences burning pain at the opening of the vagina during the initial few seconds or first minute of intercourse, and then the discomfort decreases. At its worst, a woman is unable to receive penetration due to the tight spasming of the opening of her vagina. Vaginismus, though expressed with physical symptoms, is rooted in anxiety. Unresolved vaginismus puts great pressure on both partners who experience frustration and hopelessness. A woman suffering from vaginismus experiences some of the cyclical dynamics similar to performance anxiety. There are parallels. A man caught in the trap of performance anxiety has anticipatory anxiety about erection loss. A woman with vaginismus experiences anticipatory anxiety about feeling pain, but also the failure being available for intercourse. In both cases, the more pressure she feels, the worse the condition gets. If a woman is to try to succeed by enduring great pain, the condition worsens as a self-fulfilling prophecy. The way out of this problem is through a reduction in anxiety and pressure while learning to relax. Comfort with and attitudes about sex are often problematic issues needing improvement. Whenever pain, anxiety and negativity infect a sex life, partners are at risk for developing dysfunctions including performance anxiety.

PENIS SIZE

Feeling badly about your penis and testicles is a source of negativity that may significantly contribute to performance anxiety. As briefly discussed before, because many men feel that their penises are a reflection of their masculinity, many men worry about that their penis is

> Because many men feel that their penises are a part of determining their masculinity, many men worry that their penis is not good enough.

not good

enough. In the discussion about how they feel about their penises, men commonly refer to their high school locker room as a moment when they compared their penises with others' and painfully observed that some of the other boys having larger or longer penises. Penises vary most widely when flaccid and vary much less when erect. The average penis is roughly five and six inches long. General light conversation in groups often includes jokes about how "size matters." Women have also been influenced by myths about masculinity rather than the reality. Some women have adopted an erotic interest in large penises, though in reality, sexual excitement is more about the mind and the emotions than about our genitalia. As the saying expresses it this way, "It's not about the size of the boat, rather it's about the motion of the ocean."

When we discuss matters of people, there are always those who don't fit the average. Some men have large penises and other have small penises. Some women have a preference. In cases where the female partner has a small vagina and the male partner has a large penis, painful intercourse will result. In the opposite configuration partners can make adjustments to increase their pleasure and satisfaction. Men with large penises, while having earned the envy of other men must live with difficulties that are painful. The Kama Sutra discusses the challenge for couples where genitalia size is mismatched by suggested varying positions for intercourse which use the size difference as a benefit.

> Men in porn videos and pictures are chosen especially for their large penises and are not representative of normal size.

Much penis insecurity arises from the source of young men's sexual education, mostly from porn, where men in the videos and pictures are chosen especially for having large penises and are not representative of normal size. But many men, especially those already struggling with insecurity, internalize the difference between their penis and that of the sex actor and conclude that they are woefully inadequate. Similarly, Hollywood movies and TV shows choose many actors based on their attractiveness and physical features; those actors are not representative of the average person. Think about it: for survival of the species and for the greatest genetic variety nature has designed most penises to be a good fit for most vaginas.

Men who worry often, even obsess, about their whether their male equipment is good enough are really struggling to feel good about themselves. Worrying about penises is really an expression of personal confidence and adequacy. Overwhelmingly, most penises are good enough, especially when attached to a confident man who knows how to love himself and is a skilled as well as educated lover. It is an issue of self-esteem and also anxiety. Another self-fulfilling prophecy is that if you worry that your penis is not good enough, it won't be. Penis insecurity can be a large contributor to the problem of erectile dysfunction with performance anxiety.

Non-sexual Contributing Factors

Many factors unrelated to sex are the source of negative influence. Many of them have already been explored and may be repeated here. Any negative factor, if not soothed and moderated, may fuel anxiety and distract a man by rendering his erection fragile. Throughout this course, you have been instructed to cultivate your emotional strength to reduce the influences of these factors instead of increasing their harmful influence. Stress, internalized anger, fatigue, self-hate, fear, and anxiety all contribute to being stuck in the cycle of performance anxiety.

GOAL ORIENTATION

Setting and achieving goals is good in everyday life, but they can cause trouble sexually. When we have set a goal, force and intention will be used. The best sex is free of force and goals, unless specific play is agreed to by both partners that include force, otherwise it will be negative. While attempting to succeed at maintaining an erection or producing an orgasm in either partner, having a specific goal like this reduces the overall quality of the sexual experience. If you are driving to a destination, getting there is your goal. Having a destination causes a driver to focus on the goal rather than being relaxed and enjoying the journey. Going for a ride without any destination is a more relaxed when enjoying the ride is its purpose. A sexual experience is similar. Goal orientation and the force that is used to achieve expected results places unanticipated limits on the pleasure partners experience. With a goal in mind, partners are less likely to explore, be creative and enjoy the journey. When partners focus on a goal, they are focused from intention rather than living free in relaxation.

TRYING

Worry and pressure are factors that supply with energy the gravitational pull of the performance anxiety trap. When you apply pressure to your partner she will almost always experience it as negative. It will be detrimental to your connection. Self-pressure, as we have explored, also is counterproductive; it leads away from a relaxed state and into erection loss. Another factor that gets men ensnared in the trap is the concept of "trying." When we are trying to achieve a specific outcome, force is being used. The natural you is relaxed and fully present in the moment. The natural you is not trying because trying is unnecessary for success. Instead, it is more effective to be open and fluid and flexible by responding as the moment requires, without purpose or plan, to give as the moment requires, to stay open to your experience, and love your partner; all without trying.

Trying can introduce troubles for couples who set sexual goals in their lovemaking, especially when their goals are insensitive to natural factors. A relevant dynamic lies in the difference between male and female bodies. A woman's clitoris, her chief organ for pleasure and orgasm, is not directly stimulated during intercourse because it is located outside her vagina. In a natural fact of inequality, the tip of the man's penis, the source of equal pleasure to the woman's clitoris, is stimulated during intercourse. Many couples hold the sexual value that both partners should reach orgasm during intercourse. Without her clitoris being stimulated, the achievement of her orgasm from intercourse is a difficult task. As mentioned before, most women do not orgasm during intercourse, making this challenge an unrealistic and unhealthy goal. A male partner who accepts responsibility for the achievement of this goal may have to put great pressure on himself to provide vigorous thrusting and lasting long enough under rigorous circumstances. Female partners may develop unrealistic sexual expectations. By putting pressure on themselves, men become vulnerable to the cycle of performance anxiety and the development of premature ejaculation. Penises do not work well under pressure. A better strategy that includes far less pressure is to have intercourse in a position where direct clitoral stimulation can occur with fingers or a toy. Both Tantra Yoga and Taoist sexual practices offer practices in the development of greater orgasmic capacity for both the genders.

A WORKER BEING PRODUCTIVE

A variation of trying is "Getting the job done." Our culture's history includes the value of productivity. The emphasis on work, productivity, and efficiency pervade our attitudes and language; they also creep into our bedrooms. Men, as traditional financial providers have incorporated these values into how masculinity is defined. The goal-orientation referenced earlier fits into this value. Men may view the satisfaction of their female partner as a job that needs completion. Maintaining his erection is like bringing the necessary tool for the task. Viewing sex as a job to be performed or a task needing completion injects the lack of choice, pressure and a non-playful attitude to your sex. Female partners are sensitive to the amount of connection present between her and her lover. This workman-like approach robs many female partners of the most important element of good sex. Instead, a playful, undefined, creative, and spontaneous atmosphere is more conducive to good sex.

PLAYFULNESS

Contrary to viewing sex as a kind of job consider sex as adult play instead of work. During play, the value is to have fun, to enjoy each other. Within fun is a focus on the present, the play, spontaneity, surprise, exploration, and discovery. All the facets of play encourage greater connection and relationship. Generally female partners value connection and feeling close above the physical element of sex. If closeness, connection, and fun are not part of sex, female partners become bored and disinterested. The quality of your connection with your partner is a large determinant of the excitement of sex and your ability to keep your erection.

Negative factors contribute to sexual problems and performance anxiety. Relationship difficulties, financial stress, and work stress, parenting worries all are problems that factor into erectile dysfunction in a significant way. The exercises throughout this course, if mastered, won't eliminate these problems but can give you the ability to prevent the emotional fall-out from these difficulties from invading parts of your life where they will be disruptive. Strong men and women react to a problem by making them smaller rather than making the problem bigger. Problems are reduced by calming intense negative emotions so that problems do not interfere with functioning.

MEDICATIONS

A final important element that contributes to sexual problems is medicine. Most medications are not friendly to good sex. Beware of medicine. Even if sexual side effects are not listed among a medication's published side effects, or even if the prescribing doctor is unaware of any sexual effects, nevertheless, you might consider the possibility that medicine is producing a dampening effect of your sexual experience. Better to stay fit and healthy by living a good lifestyle than by being dependent on pharmaceuticals. However, there are times when prescribed drugs are necessary and life-saving.

Among the most commonly prescribed drugs are antidepressant medications. A medicine interacts with each individual's physiology uniquely. Most antidepressants cause reduced sexual desire and make orgasm difficult to achieve. However, antidepressant medications can also reduce depressive feelings as well as anxiety. For some men, an antidepressant can offer a way out of performance anxiety. Of course Viagra, Cialis, and Levitra are designed to help sexual functioning, but some men experience a side effect of headaches that may neutralize the pleasure of sex. Strong emotions such as fear and anxiety, can override the erection-promoting effects of these medicines. Birth control pills prevent pregnancy, but they may also reduce sexual desire, thereby preventing pregnancy by reducing the frequency of sex. Blood pressure medications have a strong and negative effect on erections; prescribing doctors do not always communicate this side effect to their male patients. Heart problems and other heart medicines can also be detrimental to achieving erections. Most psychotropic medications have a dampening effect on desire and arousal. Recreational drugs including alcohol may have an initial boosting effect on sexual excitement and orgasm, but if used regularly can have the opposite result. Most recreational drugs will decrease partner sensitivity over time while also risking addiction. Alcohol, especially for older men, prevents erections and sexual functioning.

Emotional exercise 19: In your journal, write about what you learned from all of these factors that contribute to performance anxiety. Which ones have been a part of your life, relationship and development of performance anxiety? Write this in your journal. List the specific factors which have been a challenge in your life.

Sexual exercise 12: How is it going? Has sex become more positive and relaxing? How do you rate your ability to calm yourself? Is your confidence level higher than in the past? If you can answer solidly "yes," then you may allow intercourse to be unlimited, based on your own discretion when evaluating your feelings, stress level, partner connection, etc. If the conditions are not favorable, communicate this to your partner; choose intercourse only when you are confident of your success.

Let Sex Be a Strength (read together if in a relationship)

Contrary to sex being a problem, the intention is to transform sex into a strength for you and your partner. The context of your life into which the sex fits has a big impact on whether or not sex is great. Just like a sparkling jewel, if it is placed in a poor setting, it will not shine.

Here are suggestions for sexual success that will help you maintain a reliable erection by keeping the cycle of performance anxiety at bay. Some of the ideas are repeated from before, having been included in some of the exercises you have already practiced. Think of these practices not only as a way to fix performance anxiety but as a way to maintain a high-quality sex life. The first one is to make sex relaxing and playful while avoiding future-focused goals. If you and your partner have fun and feel a lot of pleasure, orgasm for both of you need not be essential. Each of you may have strong opinions about this and can be a useful discussion. However, first and foremost, make sex relaxing and playful. Enjoy a long and relaxing embrace before foreplay begins. Include romantic music, or music that is associated with fond memories to create ambiance. Experiment with altering your space by creating an interesting or new environment in which your love making can evolve.

Slow sex down. Quickies have their time and place and can be both intense and exciting, but most sex will be more pleasurable if it is slow and sensuous. Partners who have difficulty or discomfort with a slow and sensuous pace may have to learn how to calm anxious feelings. Slowing your play way down may allow both of you to be more focused on all the sensations of your touch. Raise your awareness by being attentive to each other's breathing and body movements. Such elements provide a lot of information about what your partner is feeling, and which touches are being felt as discomfort, pleasure and high pleasure. Take your time and extend the pleasure of loving touch.

Include lots of foreplay. Rushing to intercourse can be an enjoyable occasional variation, but most bodies do not get sufficiently aroused at a moment's notice and can create unanticipated problems. Alternatively, lots of foreplay gives partners plenty of time to warm up and get hot. Female partners, as a group, complain of not enough foreplay. The difference in patterns of arousal between men and women may be to blame. Men arrive at full arousal in a tiny fraction of the time it takes

> Men arrive at full arousal in a tiny fraction of the time it takes most women to reach full arousal.

most women to reach full arousal. Wanting to please their men, many women choose to engage in intercourse before they are ready. If both partners are at high excitement, the level of pleasure and satisfaction for both partners will be higher. Not only does foreplay build excitement and arousal, but it also includes many pleasurable ways to tease and stimulate. By including a lot of foreplay, you are increasing the total pleasure of a sexual session.

In line with the need for more foreplay, another beneficial adjustment is for female partners to give the signal for readiness. Consider the female partner inviting the male partner to enter her vagina. Sex need not be this way all the time, but it has important advantages. Only women know their bodies. Only women are aware of their own arousal. Only a woman knows when she is truly eager for intercourse. If she does not arrive at the place of readiness, then the sexual session may have to be fulfilling without intercourse, which can be OK. If the female partner objects at being direct about inviting intercourse, perhaps she may use a discreet agreed upon gesture to signal readiness. Sexual desire will be higher for both of you if sex is often highly satisfying. Your lovemaking will be of higher quality if intercourse is eagerly anticipated by both of you. If the female partner regularly arrives at high arousal, the male partner has more to excite him, thus helping with a solid, reliable erection. Practicing sensitivity to the female partner's arousal over time may improve the male partner's ability to read his female partner so that initiating intercourse becomes natural.

Shift your sexual loving away from intercourse and towards other ways to give and receive touch and pleasure by exploring and experimenting. Being less dependent on intercourse means that as a man, the success and pleasure of sex will be less be dependent upon your erection, so there is less pressure. Consider a common dinner plate with the main entree and several side dishes. It's good and can be satisfying but need not be the same in each meal. Sometimes a great meal can come from several really good side dishes, or having the side dishes prepared in a new and interesting way. Sex is the same. Let intercourse be less of an entree and more of a side dish while other "side dishes" are increased in importance.

Celebrate your whole bodies. Instead of focusing on your sensitive erogenous zones, such as nipples, clitoris and penis, expand your areas of interest to each other's entire body. Touch all over while learning about what feels good and why. Whole-body massages are wonderful foreplay activities and may continue throughout a sexual session. Including the whole body may also result in orgasms being more whole-body than centered in the pelvis or genitals. Your sex parts are wonderful, but you may feel much more pleasure by expanding excitement to include EVERY part of your bodies.

Couples don't talk much about sex, to their detriment. Sex is a team activity and teams function best with communication. Your relationship and your sex life will benefit from talking about sex, preferences, curiosities, sexual memories, areas of satisfaction, and new ways to explore sexual pleasure. Additionally, sexual communication also benefits the quality of your sex. While the two of you are having sex, agree to allow asking questions about sensations and pleasure. Ask for instructions. Give gently worded instructions. Talk about why you value and love your partner. Some couples have discovered excitement from talking dirty, so long as both partners enjoy it and the limitations of it are mutually understood and respected. Talk about sources of appreciation.

A variant of talk is including erotic material in your play. By using written stories and taking turns reading erotic tales to each other may have an enhancing effect on your sexual play. The stories might also provide new ways to play with each other. Unlike photos or videos, which may take partners' attention away from each other, reading to each other feels more like sharing. When imaginations are used, partners can learn about each other more.

Our sexual selves are the source of great vulnerability, so talking about sex can easily cause discomfort and hurt. Protect each other from hurt by only talking in positive ways. For instance, we can say, "Don't touch me like that," or we can say more positively, "Touching me like this feels better."

One is negative and the other is positive. Instead of talking about what you don't like or what is wrong, talk about what you do like or what will be better. Solutions are positive. Focusing on the positive is a protective measure to make sexual discussions emotionally safer.

> Protect each other from hurt by only talking in positive ways.

Words may be helpful, especially for those partners who do not share non-verbal sounds of pleasure. However expressing sounds is healthy and helpful to high quality sex. By expressing sounds of pleasure, sexual energy flow is enhanced in your body which can amplify pleasure. Sounds and noises are also more efficient communicators of your excitement and pleasure and therefore add to an upward spiral of pleasure between you. Listening to your partner's song of pleasure when it is sounds rather than words allows partners to learn of each other's level of excitement without having to think, which makes it easier for partners to stay out of their heads.

Get out of your heads! Ever notice that when you have the most fun, you have forgotten about yourself. These are times when you are not thinking. Sex, similarly, is best when touching and loving are all about sensation and not a thought is present. Place your attention lower to your body. Even though sex is highly emotional, during sex, the action is in your body. By getting out of your heads and thoughts, lovers are able to heighten their pleasure. Let your awareness be filled with sights, sounds and sensations. Feel your body and lose yourself in play. By locating your awareness in the sensations of the moment, you make possible being transported to a realm of pleasure where the whole world is just you, your Beloved and love.

The bedroom is the standard place for sex for most couples, for many good reasons. However, novelty is an important source of interest, aliveness and excitement in sex. Rearranging your bedroom may add newness and spice. If your bedroom is cluttered with items of daily living, such as piles of clothes or unfolded laundry, then your space for loving each other is littered with reminders of responsibilities, sources of tension, or triggers of resentment. A peaceful mind helps with excitement and pleasure. Consider making your bedroom more of a sacred space that supports peace of mind, being relaxed, and of being in a positive mood. Respect your love by making your bedroom beautiful and pleasing. Altering the bedroom's ambiance with scented candles, low light, relaxing sensuous music, or drapes and sheets to create a tent may offer an environment that nourishes a fantasy world away from the desire-killing effects of daily life.

The bedroom is not the only authorized location for sex. Mix it up by choosing rooms and locations (not risky, immoral, or illegal locations, please) not normally associated with sexual pleasure. Pleasing sexual interludes in non-sexual locations can add a layer of freshness that can create a powerful togetherness and a strongly positive memory. Having sex in the shower while you wash each other may combine hygiene with sexual fun, a great combination. Use the water as an instrument of pleasure, such as with a hand-held shower head that has many spray settings.

Another standard for a majority of couples is relegating sex to the final minutes of the day. This makes sense since it is one of the few times when partners are together in bed. And it is usually dark, a benefit of those partners who are uncomfortable with their bodies being revealed in the light of day. But great sex requires a lot of energy which is in low supply in the last few waking minutes of a day. Perhaps with a bit of effort and creativity, move sex to a different time of the day when you have more energy. Great sex requires great energy.

So many of us get locked into routines. Our mindset gets locked up, too. Consider possibilities you would otherwise reject by thinking deeply about how you could manifest the impossible. Think of ideas such as calling into work a bit late and enjoying sexual pleasure as your day begins or arranging to unite in the afternoon when the kids are still in school. If you have privacy, perhaps a sexy interlude before dinner and before your stomachs are full and you become tired. You might even incorporate some appetizers into your play. When your mind is open to possibilities, what seems impossible may now appear possible. Instead of saying no, say "Let's find a way."

Ancient traditions exist in which sexual practices have been honed to an art. The term "Sacred Sexuality" refers to ancient traditions of incorporating deep relaxation, reverence of life and the joining of partners in love. Both traditions of Tantra Yoga and Taoism offer sexual and meditative practices which can take your lovemaking to heights of pleasure and quality that you have never imagined. Both traditions incorporate not just great sex but also high quality of health and life. Explore these traditions, they provide practices which will help you banish anxiety and failed erections.

Emotional exercise 20: In a discussion with your partner, talk about the above-mentioned suggestions regarding a stronger sex life. Identify which suggestions the two of you can put into action.

Setting Yourself Up for Success

Escaping the cycle of performance anxiety and staying out of the trap is the same process as loving yourself. Love is experienced, expressed, and given in the numerous ways we have explored. By practicing all the ways of loving, you will strengthen your ability to stay free of emotionally-based erectile dysfunction, but while doing so you will give yourself a better quality of life.

The theme of loving yourself has been a thread running through this entire course. Forgiving yourself for past mistakes and failures, for living a life with pain, and of past regrets will gradually free you so that no obstacles stand in the way of a life with satisfying love and passion. Being a good friend to yourself means always putting yourself in a good position. The work of being emotionally disciplined in your choices is hard at first but rewards you later on as you feel better and better. By operating with care and living from internal calmness you will prevent making missteps that result in self-anger, a new rise of anxiety along with a downward emotional spiral. Instead, treat yourself and your well-being with the care that demonstrates that you are valuable. More often than not, delayed gratification, a willingness to tolerate some discomfort by putting off the fulfillment of desires, is a choice to love yourself and create a good, strong life.

Setting yourself up for success is accomplished by building a strong emotional foundation. The high quality of your life helps you to be a good lover because your sexuality is holistic, it is influenced by every part of yourself and your life. The quality of your love relationship has a huge impact on you and your success. By treating your partner as very important and with great care, you give her your best love and you get to spend time with a happy partner. As her male partner, you not only benefit from the pride that she is well, but loving her well also reinforces your confidence. Stay open to your partner so that she may join you in being a team for continued sexual success. The two of you are in this together. If you feel alone in a problem, then greater openness and a strengthened connection are needed.

If you experience a relapse in the form of a failed or disappointing erection, don't panic. By relaxing, you have the power to repair a sexual session or be ready to succeed in your next sexual opportunity. If fear or anxiety is present, you may switch to non-intercourse pleasuring while you calm yourself. Remain open to life and your partner. You now have all the tools to succeed. Daily practice is required. Don't give up. As a man, you don't need to be perfect, you need to be human.

Sexual exercise 13: Trust yourself and your awareness of your own emotional, energetic and physical limitations. Continue to practice relaxation. Within your sex life, maintain the practices that allow for relaxed togetherness. If you have moments when your penis is not erect, put the experience in reverse by engaging in less pressure-filled activities until you are more relaxed and more aroused. Your value is not determined by the presence of an erection. Trust your love for yourself and your partner when you have an erection and even when you don't.

For more than 25 years Andrew Aaron, LICSW has specialized in marriage counseling and sex therapy. He has devoted the focus of his career on helping individuals and couples love more effectively. Recently he has been featured on a weekly hour long radio program responding to callers' questions about love relationships and sex. He is also a contributor to national online publications

9. Reflect on your emotions..40
10. The self-fulfilling prophecy....................................43
11. Dealing with feeling to create repair........................48
12. Relaxed focus on the pelvis.....................................49
13. Connecting anxiety and arousal...............................51
14. Putting emotions into words....................................58
15. Importance of relationship connection.....................66
16. The partner's experience and feelings.....................74
17. Developing emotional strengths..............................80
18. Eliminating negative tendencies.............................85
19. Factors that contribute..104
20. Suggestions for great sex......................................112

Sexual exercises
  1. Discontinue intercourse...4
  2. Masturbation...8
  3. Erections during partner sex.................................10
  4. Redefining a "good enough" erection..................14
  5. The long embrace..15
  6. Daily observations of arousal, erections..............22
  7. Checking in on intercourse prohibition...............31
  8. Erections during together times..........................37
  9. Re-evaluate intercourse.......................................51
  10. Lengthen intercourse?.......................................66
  11. Evaluate your state of readiness.........................86
  12. Evaluating your confidence..............................104
  13. Trusting your sexual self..................................113

Made in the USA
Middletown, DE
07 August 2021